CHINA: BIOETHICS, TRUST, AND THE CHALLENGE OF THE MARKET

AF840838

Philosophy and Medicine

VOLUME 96

Founding Co-Editor
Stuart F. Spicker

Senior Editor

H. Tristram Engelhardt, Jr., *Department of Philosophy, Rice University, and Baylor College of Medicine, Houston, Texas*

Associate Editor

Lisa M. Rasmussen, *Department of Philosophy, University of North Carolina at Charlotte, Charlotte*

ASIAN STUDIES IN BIOETHICS AND THE PHILOSOPHY OF MEDICINE 6

Series Editor

Ruiping Fan, *Department of Public & Social Administration, City University of Hong Kong, Hong Kong*

Editorial Advisory Board

Kazumasa Hoshino, *Kyoto Women's University, Kyoto, Japan*
Shui Chuen Lee, *National Central University, Chung-li, Taiwan*
Ping-Cheung Lo, *Hong Kong Baptist University, Hong Kong*
Ren-Zong Qiu, *Chinese Academy of Social Sciences, Beijing, China*

For other titles published in this series, go to
www.springer.com/series/6414

CHINA: BIOETHICS, TRUST, AND THE CHALLENGE OF THE MARKET

Edited by

JULIA TAO

City University of Hong Kong, China

Springer

Editor
Julia Tao
City University of Hong Kong
China
sajulia@cityu.edu.hk

ISBN: 978-90-481-7714-1 e-ISBN: 978-1-4020-6757-0

© 2008 Springer Science+Business Media B.V.
Softcover reprint of the hardcover 1st edition 2008
No part of this work may be reproduced, stored in a retrieval system, or transmitted in any form or by any means, electronic, mechanical, photocopying, microfilming, recording or otherwise, without written permission from the Publisher, with the exception of any material supplied specifically for the purpose of being entered and executed on a computer system, for exclusive use by the purchaser of the work.

Printed on acid-free paper

9 8 7 6 5 4 3 2 1

springer.com

Acknowledgments

On behalf of all the contributors, I wish to express deep appreciation to the Governance in Asia Research Centre (GARC) of the City University of Hong Kong for its support and financial assistance to the research project "Health Care, Market, Morality, and Resources of Traditional Culture," from which the papers in this volume are derived. Appreciation should also be conveyed to the Institute of Medical Humanities, Shandong University, Jinan, PRC, Journal of Medicine and Philosophy, and International Studies in Philosophy and Medicine, who were co-sponsors of the research as well as co-organizers with GARC of an international conference based on this project on 27–28 June 2006 at the Institute of Medical Humanities of Shandong University, and a follow-up conference on "The Role and the Challenges of the Market in Health Care Reform: Cross-cultural Perspectives" held at City University of Hong Kong on 2 July 2005.

The project team is deeply indebted to Professor H. Tristram Engelhardt, Jr. who has been a prime mover and an invaluable source of inspiration to the project. The support and advice offered by Professor Xiaoyang Chen and Professor Yongfu Cao of the Institute of Medical Humanities, Shandong University, in the implementation of the research and organization of the international conference in Jinan were germane to the success enjoyed by the project. We are also very grateful to Dr. Jeremy Garrett, Dr. Aaron Hinkley, and Ms Virginia Chan for their professional assistance to the project and to the preparation of this book manuscript for publication.

A final note of appreciation also goes to Lakshmi Praba. A and to Springer for their excellent support in the production of this book volume *China: Bioethics, Trust, and the Challenge of the Market.*

Julia Tao, Ph.D.
Professor, Department of Public and Social Administration Director
Governance in Asia Research Centre
City University of Hong Kong, Hong Kong

Contents

Contributors

Yongfu Cao
Professor in the Department of Medical Ethics, Medical Ethics Institute, Medical School, Shandong University Shandong Medical College, China
cyongfu@sdu.edu.cn

Xiaoyang Chen
Professor in the Department of Medical Ethics, Medical School of Shandong University, Shandong University Medical College, Shandong, China
chenxy@sdu.edu.cn

Zhizheng Du
Dalian Medical University, PRC
duzhi@mail.dlptt.ln.cn

H. Tristram Engelhardt, Jr., M.D., Ph.D.
Professor of Philosophy, Rice University, and Professor Emeritus, Baylor College of Medicine
htengelh@rice.edu

Ruiping Fan, Ph.D.
Associate Professor in the Department of Public and Social Administration, City University of Hong Kong, Hong Kong, PRC
safan@cityu.edu.hk

Frederic J. Fransen, Ph.D.
Liberty Fund, Inc., Indianapolis, IN USA
ffransen@libertyfund.org

Jeremy Garrett, M.A., Ph.D.
Assistant Professor in the Department of Philosophy, California State University, Sacramento, Sacramento, California
garrettj@rice.edu

Aaron E. Hinkley, Ph.D.
Candidate in the Department of Philosophy, Rice University, and Senior Managing Editor of the *Journal of Medicine and Philosophy*
hinkley@rice.edu

Justin Ho, Ph.D.
Candidate in the Department of Philosophy, Rice University, and Assistant Managing Editor of the *Journal of Medicine and Philosophy*
justinho@rice.edu

Linying Hu
Director of the Department of Medical Ethics, Peking University, Health Science Center
hulinying@bjmu.edu.cn

Ana Iltis, Ph.D.
Assistant Professor in the Center for Health Care Ethics, Saint Louis University, Saint Louis, Missouri, USA
iltisas@slu.edu

Benfu Li
Director of the Department of Medical Ethics, Peking University, Health Science Center
libenfubest@126.com

Yanwen Li
Professor in the Department of Medical Ethics, Medical School of Shandong University, Shandong University Medical College, Shandong, China

Ren-Zong Qiu
Professor in the Institute of Philosophy, Chinese Academy of Social Sciences, Beijing, PRC, China
rzq@chinaphs.org

Xiuqin Shen
Professor in the Department of Medical Ethics, Medical School of Shandong University, Shandong University Medical College, Shandong, China
xiuqin@sdu.edu.cn

Julia Tao, Ph.D.
Associate Professor in the Department of Public and Social Administration, City University of Hong Kong
sajulia@cityu.edu.hk

Yunling Wang
Professor in the Department of Medical Ethics, Medical Ethics Institute, Medical School, Shandong University Shandong Medical College, China
wangyl@sdu.edu.cn

Tongwei Yang
Professor in the Department of Medical Ethics, Medical School of Shandong University, Shandong University Medical College, Shandong, China
yangtw@sdu.edu.cn

Li Yanwen
Professor in the Department of Medical Ethics, Medical Ethics Institute, Medical School, Shandong University Shandong Medical College, China
lywtv@yahoo.com.cn

Linjuan Zheng
Professor in the Department of Medical Ethics, Medical Ethics Institute, Medical School, Shandong University Shandong Medical College, China
zhenglinjuan@sdu.edu.cn

Part I
Introduction: Trust, the Market, and Bioethics

The Bioethics of Trust

Julia Tao

Health care reform in China is at a crossroads. The moral and policy challenges of improving the equity, quality and sustainability of the country's health system are pressing. The health of the society is declining and the voice of discontent is rising. Should China develop a market-based health care system with private hospitals and physicians in private practice, and in which health care services must increasingly be paid by those who consume them? Or should China adopt the social democratic model and establish a health care which provides free basic health care as a right for all citizens?

There are evidences that market forces have made the health system generally much more receptive to change and innovation in China in the recent years. This has created a wider range and better quality of service, while also bringing about more choice and greater dynamism in the system. But at the same time, the market law of demand and supply is excluding millions of Chinese people from access to basic health care (China Development Review, 2005). The Chinese health care system was ranked 188 out of 191 countries in terms of distributional and financial equity in the 2000 WHO report. In terms of overall health achievement, China ranked 144. In 2003, less that half of the urban inhabitants were covered by medical insurance (see Qiu in this volume). At the same time, the profit principle is also undermining the medical ethics which defines the patient–physician relationship. The lack of effective regulation of the health care market have led to serious abuses such as bribes for better services, improper use or over-use of drugs and technological interventions, issues of cost control and rapid increase in spending of health care. Increasingly health care is being turned into an exchange commodity, while its social purpose and welfare function are being eroded.

In fact there are growing concerns that the growth of private sector in health-care provision may lead to rapid cost escalation, reduced equity, and poor quality or inappropriate health care (Bennett, McPake, & Mills, 1997; Benson, 2001; Berman, 1997; Chakraborty & Frick, 2002). These concerns raise serious questions

---

J. Tao, Ph.D.
Department of Public and Social Administration, City University of Hong Kong
e-mail: sajulia@cityu.edu.hk

J. Tao (ed.), *China: Bioethics, Trust, and the Challenge of the Market*,
© Springer Science+Business Media B.V. 2008

about whether China should accept the market solution as the model of its health care reform.

A social democratic model of health care system is committed to equal access to basic health care for all based on an egalitarian ideology. Health care is a public good and should be provided and financed by the State. A public health care system fulfils an important welfare function, and promotes solidarity and mutual responsibility in society. But such a model also raises serious questions of sustainability because of ever rising health care expenditures, rapidly increasing proportion of the elderly in the population, and escalating costs of modern medical technologies. An egalitarian model of health care is also confronted with problems of moral and political hazards (see Englehardt in this volume), lack of incentives for dynamic innovation and weak personal responsibility for health.

A third possible solution which has been suggested is the introduction of mandatory individual savings account which one finds in the Singaporean system. It is a model recommended for China on the ground that its family- and savings- oriented commitments can encourage personal responsibility for health, avoid moral hazards, support family mutual help and reduce government economic burden. Moreover, the system is considered by their advocate to be consistent with traditional Confucian family values. But there are also serious doubts about the Singaporean solution for China. As a developing country with a huge gap between the rich and the poor, reducing government expenditure and transferring the financial burden to the individual will result in a large proportion of the population not being able to receive the health care they need. Some would argue that a Confucian *ren* ethic would in fact justify an expansion, rather than a reduction, of government's role in health care to look after the welfare of the people (see Du in this volume).

Some recent studies on Southeast Asia also suggest that privatization might lead to cost escalation (Ramesh, 2004). In the past decades, many Southeast Asian countries have embarked on privatization of healthcare provision, hoping that private sector will lighten the government's burden. The resulting shift in the relationship between public–private mix and access to healthcare suggest the expansion of the role of the private providers is achieved at retarded growth for the health system in general. Evidences show that the slack created by governments' retreat from health care provision has not been filled by the private sector. This has curtailed the population's access to healthcare.

There is no denying that competition among providers improves services at the level of individual patients. But costs to the society as a whole may be high. As scholars have pointed out, in the healthcare sector, unlike most goods and services, competition among multitude of providers may promote duplication of expensive equipments and services and misplaced emphasis on frills, the combined results of which may be higher rather than lower expenditures (Ramesh & Wu, 2007). For the same reason, a universal health insurance program may also not be a viable option for financing healthcare in developing countries. The third party payment could induce moral hazard problems since consumer demand is no longer constrained by prices. A government-run insurance scheme may further exacerbate the problem as there would be no pressures to control costs because of the lack of profit motive.

A recent study on the impacts of public–private mix on national health system by comparing health policy reform in four Southeast Asian countries found that the public sector's dominance of healthcare provision is a key reason for maintaining healthcare costs at a modest level (Ramesh & Wu, 2007). Experience such as that of Thailand is particularly worth noting. It has shown that public sector dominance in health care provision together with the use of capitation fees to providers is the key to success in preventing cost escalation in health care.

Which should be the way forward for China? It is clear that which ever model China is to develop, the choice must be able to respond adequately to the moral and policy challenges of quality of care, equity in access and long-term sustainability. Debates on the form of the extent of private sector participation in healthcare must consider more critically the interlinkages between provision and financing while designing reform. Success of reform will depend on government's ability to restrain the profit-maximizing urges of the providers to overcharge and over treat on the one hand, and to control corruption, incompetence and bureaucratic conflicts on the other hand. Chinese moral traditions and cultural values, as demonstrated in several essays in this volume, can offer rich intellectual resources to construct an ethical framework for the reform process to meet the challenge of the new century.

We wish to acknowledge our deep appreciation to the Institute of Medical Ethics at the Medical School of Shandong University; International Studies in Philosophy and Medicine; Journal of Medicine and Philosophy; and Governance in Asia Research Centre at the City University of Hong Kong for their generous funding and research support. We also wish to register a special note of thanks to Aaron Hinkley, Justin Ho, Jeremy Garrett and Virginia Chan for their editing support and general assistance to the authors of this volume. As always, Professor Tris Engelhardt has been a valuable source of inspiration. We have benefited immensely from both our agreements and our disagreements. They are importantly the sources of our dynamism.

References

An evaluation of and recommendations on the reforms of the health system in China (executive summary). (2005). *China Development Review. New York: St. Martin's Press, 7*(1), 1–24.

Bennett, S., McPake, B., & Mills, A. (Eds.). (1997). The public/private mix debate in healthcare. *Private healthcare providers in developing countries: Serving the public interest* (pp.1–18). Zed Books.

Benson, J. S. (2001). The impact of privatization on access in Tanzania. *Social Science and Medicine, 52*, 1903–1915.

Berman, P. (1997). Supply-side approaches to optimizing private health care sector growth. In W. Newbrander (Ed.), *Private health sector in Asia: Issues and implications.* London: Routledge.

Chakraborty, S., & Frick, K. (2002). Factors influencing private health provider's technical quality of care for acute respiratory infections among under – five children in rural West Bengal, India. *Social Science Medicine, 55*, 1579–1587.

Ramesh, M. (2004). Social Policy in East and Southeast Asia: Education, health, housing, and income maintenance. London: Routledge Curzon.

Ramesh, M., & Wu, X. (2007, January). Realigning public–private mix in healthcare: Comparative health policies in southeast Asia. Paper presented at the Governance in Asia Research Centre, City University of Hong Kong.

Chinese Health Care Policy: An Introduction to the Moral Challenges

H. Tristram Engelhardt, Jr. and Aaron E. Hinkley

1 Taking Finitude Seriously in a Chinese Cultural Context

Across the world, health care policy is a moral and political challenge. Few want to die young or to suffer, yet not all the money in the world can deliver physical immortality or a life free of suffering. In addition, health care needs differ. As a result, unless a state coercively forbids those with the desire and means to buy better basic health care to do so, access to medicine will be unequal. No country can afford to provide all with the best of care. In countries such as China, there are in addition stark regional differences in the quality and availability of health care, posing additional challenges to public policy-making. Further, in China as elsewhere, the desire to lower morbidity and mortality risks has led to ever more resources being invested in health care. When such investment is supported primarily by funds derived from taxation, an increasing burden is placed on a country's economy. This is particularly the case as in China with its one-child policy, where the proportion of the elderly population consuming health care is rising.

These policy challenges are compounded by moral diversity. De facto, humans do not share one morality. Instead, they rank cardinal human goods and right-making conditions in different orders, often not sharing an affirmation of the same goods or views of the right. Thus, depending on how one orders such cardinal moral concerns as liberty, equality, prosperity, and security, one will affirm a social-democratic policy or a one-party capitalist polity such as Singapore. In this regard, at the beginning of the twenty first century, China stands at the crossroads. It can affirm a social democratic ideology as the basis for a health care policy and seek to sustain a health care system as in most of Europe and in Canada. Such a policy choice will send China down the road toward the financial challenges of the social-welfare state: the social-democratic welfare state does not appear to be economically sustainable. Or, instead, China can follow a model based on Confucian values, as one finds in Singapore, where by ranking security first, prosperity second, liberty third, and

H.T. Engelhardt Jr., M.D., Ph.D.
Professor of Philosophy, Rice University, and Professor Emeritus, Baylor College of Medicine
e-mail: htengelh@rice.edu

J. Tao (ed.), *China: Bioethics, Trust, and the Challenge of the Market*,

© Springer Science+Business Media B.V. 2008

equality last, a policy of compelling each to save for his own health care (along with a back-up catastrophic health care policy) can be pursued. This choice will not only accumulate capital, but it can be structured to support Confucian family values. For example, by allowing a transfer of funds among family members, Singapore affirms values and a view of flourishing in greater agreement with preponderant East Asian values.

This choice of a health care policy for China must be made in light of the emerging economic and health policy data that demonstrate the obvious: the ideology of social-democratic approaches presumes that one can do the impossible. Given the finitude of human life, the intractability of human suffering, and the limitations of human resources, one cannot provide all persons with equal care and the best care to meet their health care needs, much less meet all of their desires. Providing the best care to all is incompatible with the human condition. Given this circumstance, one must appreciate the challenges to contemporary health care policy. To begin with, even insurance-supported health care entitlements generate a moral hazard: once an entitlement is in place, people tend to exploit it, even when the costs are high and the benefits low. In addition, contemporary welfare systems are now exposed to the demographic hazard: in developing countries there is an ever-increasing proportion of the population that is aged and that consumes relatively high amounts of expensive care, while there is an ever-decreasing proportion of the population that is young, healthy, willing and able to pay the taxes to support this care. This demographic hazard is a major challenge to China, which has become old before it has become rich. Despite this demographic hazard, in welfare states there is the additional political hazard such that, once health care is seen to be the province of the government, politicians then try to advance their political careers by promising entitlements that future politicians may find difficult if not impossible to fund. Welfare approaches to health care combine all of these difficulties with a hazard to virtue by discouraging an internal locus of responsibility (i.e., the responsibility of individuals and families to care for their own) in favor of an external locus of responsibility (i.e., the responsibility is shifted to the society or the state). Last but not least, there is the philosophical hazard that, despite a plurality of moral visions, there is the temptation coercively to impose one particular view of justice and fairness on all (e.g., as in Canada's prohibition of a private tier of health care). There is no one canonical secular moral vision or secular bioethics (Engelhardt, 2006).

In the face of these hazards and given the cultural context of China, the question is whether China will embrace a Western social-democratic welfare approach to health care policy (one likely to impose considerable burdens on the economic development on which large sections of its population depend in order to achieve an acceptable level of resources), or whether China will embrace a policy approach such as Singapore's, which coerces persons to save funds for health care within a family-affirming policy that avoids much of the moral, demographic, and political hazards besetting Western social democracies. In addition, the Singaporean model of mandatory health savings accounts offers the allure of affirming a locus of responsibility internal to the family, while leaving individuals and families wide choices regarding their own health care choices. The decision between a health care policy grounded in a Western social-democratic welfare ideology and one grounded in East Asian-Confucian mores exemplified by the Singaporean approach will likely have dramatic implications for China's long-term economic future. Social welfare approaches will very likely significantly constrain China's economic growth. The latter is likely to support the possibility that China can become the leading culture in the twenty first century.

The development of a market-based health care system with private hospitals and physicians in private practice, and in which health care services must increasingly be paid by those who consume them, poses particular public-relations challenges against the background of recent Chinese history. Until only a few years ago, most individuals in China had access to only very low-technology health care. Even when this health care was of a low quality, it may have been provided with dedication. In addition, broad health care benefits were secured through low-cost, high-yield public health interventions, which not only remain in place, but which have increased in scope. With the availability of high-cost diagnostic and therapeutic interventions, many may not appreciate that the new benefits now being offered, which all may not be able to purchase, nevertheless exist in a system that has generally improved the quality of health care. This state of affairs is then set within a market economy, which rather than asserting an ideology of equality and welfare instead emphasizes the benefits that emerge in a system driven by profit (e.g., of medical innovation). However beneficial the market, the market suffers in comparison with the allure of promises of a social-democratic moral perspective, even if these promises cannot be met.

When the defenders of the market correctly emphasize its benefits, the market may still be faulted as lacking in altruism, even in the face of the market's considerable contributions to society. There is an immediate allure to the promise of equal access to the best of care for all, even when realistically this cannot be secured. More moral fortitude and honesty are required in coming to terms with the challenges of the human condition. The introduction of the market in China also suffers under the burden of a nostalgia for a simpler past when there was less concern for (and less possibility of) profit. Against the background of this past when physicians often needed to invest considerable energies to secure minimally appropriate care for their patients, and in which the status of physicians was not tied to financial success (and when there were fewer goods and services to be purchased through financial success), the contemporary moral status of physicians may appear inadequate and their dedication superficial. As with many crises, when resources are limited and challenges considerable, there is a sense of community and often a special dedication to virtue, which abate when the crisis abates. Now, in a period of relative luxury, such community feeling and professional dedication to virtue may not be as salient.

This complex state of affairs that places a burden on the acceptance of market solutions, which is made worse in China by the circumstance that patients in public hospitals may often only be able to secure better basic care for themselves and their family by offering unofficial payments (i.e., bribes or "red packets"), and where physicians with greater skill may only receive compensation for the superior skill they can offer by accepting such illegal payments. Given artificial constraints on physician remuneration, and given the lack of such restraints on profits from the prescription of drugs or the use of high-technology diagnostic and therapeutic interventions, such drugs may be over-prescribed or even wrongly prescribed, and such technological interventions over-used or wrongly used. Given that these abuses have arisen just as the market offers greater rewards for better services and greater skills, these abuses are often attributed to the influence of the market rather than to a set of distorting governmentally imposed, low salary scales, perverse bonus systems, and misguiding regulations. Although such abuses as bribes for better services and the improper use or over-use of drugs and technological interventions are the result of misconceived governmental policies and the failure of the rule of law, they are often laid at the foot of the market, because they are in part motivated by profit. Only recently has there been a large range of goods and services to be acquired through ill-gotten funds. Thus, as it frames its health care policy for the future, China will need not only to look at the long-range promises of such approaches as offered by Singapore, but China will need as well forthrightly to come to terms with past and current abuses.

2 The Essays: Many Voices Regarding China

This volume's first section explores contemporary Chinese health care policy. It does so in light of China's turn to the market and the benefits from the market that have transformed China over the last third of a century. China is now confronted with the challenge of completing its transformation into a market economy, including facing the implications of these developments for health care. It must also draw the difficult lessons from the financial challenges threatening the welfare state. In order for China to claim the twenty first century, it will need to find a different, perhaps nearly uniquely East Asian approach to health care policy. This section begins with "Towards a Confucian Approach to Health Care Allocation in China: A Dynamic Geography" by Yongfu Cao, Yunling Wang, and Lingjuan Zheng, who argue that, since the beginning of the economic reforms in China in 1978, there have been substantial changes in China's health care system, raising cardinal moral and policy concerns. Their focus is on traditional Confucian values and the role they should play in China's future health care system. The authors argue that, to appreciate the transformation that has taken place in China's health care system along with the market reforms since the late 1970s and the 1980s, one must first understand the health care system that was put into place after 1949. This health care system consisted of several strata of health care coverage. There was the provision of health care for industrial workers, along with some free health care in the urban areas, albeit for the most part very minimal health care, in many rural areas. The health care coverage for industrial workers was intended to cover job-related injuries and illnesses. The free health care system was for employees working in public institutions as well as university students. Cooperative health care in rural areas was intended to serve all the members of the community and was based on mutual cooperation and traditional Chinese values. Healthy members of the community were made to contribute monetarily to cover the health care costs of members of the community in need of health care. These costs were in part supported through government subsidies. Much of such care was of a very limited and very basic nature.

According to the authors, this health care system embodied Confucianism's moral values as exemplified by the maxim of "people as the foremost; the benevolent man loving others; and medical treatment as the principle and humanity as the method." This health care system claimed to promote the development of health care in China. At the same time, this system of free health care was severely limited despite its inflated claims. In urban areas people frequently over-utilized the health care services because they did not bear the costs of those services. Furthermore, given a very local level of management, the quality and access to services varied significantly from place to place. Also, since the system of free health care was limited to those working in publicly owned enterprises, state organizations, and other public institutions, the quantity and quality of health care in China for this reason varied dramatically. As a result of economic reforms and the growth of individual, private, and foreign-owned businesses, matters became even more complex. Moreover, the system of cooperative health care in the rural areas lacked stability due to its dependence on the decisions of individual leaders in individual towns made at particular times.

The authors argue that, as a result of the market reforms in society generally, reforms of China's health care system have become necessary. The necessary reforms, they argue, must place more emphasis on traditional Chinese, particularly Confucian, principles such as benevolence. As the authors observe, recent changes have been limited in their scope. Urban health care reforms have centered on adding private commercial insurance and medical savings accounts as supplements to the previous system. The authors call for the continued supplementation of the old system with commercial health insurance in urban areas and the rebuilding of cooperative health care systems in rural areas. This supplementation of the health care system with private commercial insurance plans is held to be necessary because, according to the authors, 70.3% of Chinese people do not have any form of institutionalized health care funding (79.0% in rural areas and 44.8% in urban). The authors argue that further reform would require the government of the People's Republic of China to spend funds to create additional hospitals and to provide health care assistance for the poor. Nevertheless, given the demographic hazard facing China (fewer young to support ever more elderly), future health care policy will need to avoid the pitfalls of the welfare state (e.g., through health savings accounts).

The second contribution to this section, "Trust is the Core of the Doctor–Patient Relationship: From the Perspective of Traditional Chinese Medical Ethics" by Benfu Li and Linying Hu, is concerned that in the market the physician/patient relationship is shaped by the laws of supply and demand. They register the changes brought by the market. With the advent of market reforms, the physician/patient relationship has changed (e.g., some patients can now afford to purchase better basic care). Li and Hu argue that, along with the various reforms taking place in the Chinese health care system, there should be a return to traditional Confucian medical ethics in order to build, if not restore, trust within the physician/patient relationship. In Chinese this Confucian concept of trust is termed *cheng xin*. *Cheng* by itself has the meaning of the virtue of an individual moral agent, while *xin* implies socialized moral actions. Therefore, to have *cheng xin* implies that a person is trusted by others in the community because of his personal integrity. The authors argue that this concept has an important role to play in the physician/patient relationship in China.

According to the authors, a basic principle of traditional Chinese medical ethics has been "medicine as benevolent cause", supporting a view that physicians should try their best even when there is even little hope of success, act with little regard for their own personal safety, and sometimes even be willing to give up their own life in order to save the patient. Because the disparity in knowledge places the patient in a position inferior to the physician, traditional Chinese medical ethics demands that the physician protect the interests of the patient and support that trust necessary for the achievement of medicine's goals. Traditional Chinese medical ethics places emphasis on professional duties, including the physicians' obligations to cultivate a morality appropriate to the medical profession. This moral perspective carries with it corresponding rules of conduct for patients. Traditional Chinese medical ethics seeks to nurture a spirit of selflessness. But, as the authors acknowledge, these moral considerations must be set within the over-all context of the Chinese healthcare system.

Xiaoyong Chen, Tongwei Yang, and Xiuqin Shen in the next contribution, "Medical Resources, Market and Development of Private-Run Hospitals in China", argue that, although medical resources are often considered a public good, in reality medical resources are both a public good and a private good. Their paper shows how by failing to appreciate that medicine is also a private good, some non-market-oriented elements of Chinese health care policy have morally distorted the provision of health care. This is the case despite the trend in the People's Republic of China toward privatizing public utilities including both health care service providers and hospitals so that the market has the opportunity to supply a higher quality of health care. Private hospitals have been able to make up for some of the failures of public health care providers by providing consumers with a broader spectrum of choices, more opportunities for care, and better basic care. The competition between public and private hospitals has helped improve services, thus lowering morbidity and mortality for patients in public hospitals as well as in private hospitals. Market forces have made private hospitals generally much more receptive to change and innovation, thus creating a wider range and better quality of services. Such positive impacts of private health care establishments will likely continue to contribute increasingly to the quality of health care in mainland China.

Chen et al. provide a picture of the current complex state of affairs. When the People's Republic of China was founded in 1949, there were physicians in private practice, as well as privately owned and operated hospitals. However, this phenomenon gradually disappeared by the end of the 1960s, especially during the Cultural Revolution. The result was a period in which the quality of health care ceased to develop in step with technological developments globally. In recent years, technological development has been dramatic; care in many areas has achieved the best standards of a first-world country. Since market reforms have been introduced in China beginning in the 1980s, private hospitals have re-opened in China. Currently there are 1,500 private hospitals in the People's Republic of China. Yet, there are still more than 70,000 state-owned hospitals. The bed use rate in private hospitals at 50.6% is lower than that of state-owned hospitals at 64.6%. The general satisfaction rate at private clinics (76.7%) and private hospitals (72.7%) is higher than at their public counterparts: 54.4% for hospitals and 64.9% for clinics. According to one source sited by the authors, the cause of dissatisfaction in public health care institutions is most commonly "ineffective treatment" which accounts for 46% of the dissatisfaction, while "expensive medical cost" accounts for only 31%. According to the authors, private hospitals remain at a disadvantage in China. First, they have difficulty in being accepted as hospitals designated for treatment by health insurance policies, despite the wishes of patients in the matter. Moreover, private hospitals have higher operational costs because of unfavorable tax policies. Many private hospitals are not competitive because they are small scale with simple structures, possess a small market-share, are limited in the total medical services they can provide, and often lack the personnel and technology that public hospitals possess. Lastly, some private hospitals are frequently short of talented staff because of a lack of opportunity for research and medical education.

For private hospitals to compete with public hospitals in China, they must offer a broader range of medical services. Private hospitals will also need to move towards a higher standard of competency for their physicians and staff. This accounts for why most patients in most areas resort to public care for cardiovascular care. To improve this situation, impediments need to be removed from investing in and developing new private hospitals. In particular, the authors argue that private hospitals should be treated the same as public hospitals and that institutional barriers that block their development should be dismantled, particularly the tax policies that favor public health care institutions. For instance, there is a five-percent business volume tax levied on private hospitals. Without removing this tax, there cannot be fair competition between private and public hospitals. Moreover, for this to happen, the government would need to allow tax deductions to private hospitals not available to other private businesses for "those expenditures, which aim to (a) improve patients' medical treatment conditions, (b) prevent epidemics, and (c) reduce the medical expenses of impoverished patients." (ms. 8).

In the last contribution to this section, "China, Beware: What American Health Care Has to Learn from Singapore", H. Tristram Engelhardt, Jr., reminds the reader that the market is not everything , and that sustainable health care policy requires rule of law and the absence of distorting governmental policies. Engelhardt contends that what the market can do best is to allow individuals freely to collaborate, with the result that the market can create wealth, produce innovation, and distribute services.

He argues further that, as China moves towards a more market-oriented economy, it should avoid the mistakes made by the United States and Western Europe, which have failed to develop a sustainable approach to financing health care: health care expenditures have risen absolutely and as a percentage of the gross domestic product (the demographic hazard), while unfunded entitlements to health care have been created for a growing elderly population (the political hazard). A root of this difficulty, according to Engelhardt, has been an egalitarian ideology combined with a health insurance program and a welfarist approach. He argues that dynamic and innovative health care will always be inegalitarian. Freedom and creativity undermine equality. Attempts to equalize health care systems in the social democracies have generally leveled down the quality and quantity of health care service that consumers are able to purchase in the market. Such approaches, he argues, contrast with the family- and savings-oriented commitments of Singaporean health care policy. Health care savings accounts, unlike social-democratic welfare approaches, encourage responsible health care decisions (avoiding the moral hazard), finance health care without drawing on the funds of others (avoiding the demographic hazard), prevent politicians from promising unfunded health care entitlements (avoiding the political hazard), encourage an internal locus of responsibility (avoiding the hazard to virtue), and protect against the imposition of one moral view on unconsenting others, as if it were the one secular, moral, canonical view (avoiding the philosophical hazard).

The second section opens with "Confucian Foundations of Trust and Responsibility" by Julia Tao. In her rich study, Tao explores the goal of humanizing the market through elements of the Confucian concept of trust so as to create a responsible context for the private provision of health care. According to Tao, there are both those who claim market forces erode trust and those who claim that market competition has enhanced trust. To make sense of these two divergent views on the relationship of the market to trust, Tao creatively analyses the concept of trust by distinguishing among three orders of trust. These three orders or types of trust are paternalistic trust or first-order trust, strategic trust or second-order trust, and moralistic trust or third-order trust. Paternalistic trust, so she argues, is trust directed to persons. It is grounded in the asymmetrical power relationship between the one who trusts and the person trusted. It is the basis of traditional medical ethics. This form of trust takes into account the unequal power status of the physician and the patient. It depends on the benevolence of the physician. Strategic trust is second-order trust. It places emphasis on the procedural dimension of trust. Trust in this instance is not placed in individuals, but instead in institutions, laws, and their procedures. Trust in such cases need have no particular moral content. Or to put matters differently, the content is acquired through the instrumental goals that move one to trust others. In this context, a framework of laws and institutions will establish a rule of law that gives space for various incentives for people to act according to their own interests. People trust others not because of any quality of the other person but because of institutional structures in place that make it in everyone's best interest to keep their word. According to Tao, strategic trust involves an abstraction from personal trust, a movement from trust in other persons to trust in abstract rules and laws.

Moralistic trust constitutes the symbolic dimension of trust. As Tao argues, trust is here a moral good that sustains a culture of trust in the community. Moralistic trust treats others as if they were trustworthy in order to bind a community. Tao further argues that a society that has rule of law where citizens are autonomous, where markets are reliable, and where there is an adequate health care system, requires all three orders of trust. As she notes, within Confucian philosophy there is an emphasis on the value of trust. The moral ideal of *ren*, humanity, love, or benevolence, marks out a place for trust in Confucian moral considerations. Tao then demonstrates how Confucian thought supports all three varieties of trust. Moreover, she concludes that moralistic trust is not essential to the practice of medicine, but is an essential feature of medicine itself because as a common good it is an expression of symbolic trust.

The next contribution to this section, "The Pursuit of an Efficient, Sustainable Health Care System in China: The Role of Health Care Organizations" by Ana Iltis, examines the role that health care organizations, with institutional moral integrity, could play in Chinese health care reform. Health care organizations, hospitals, and other establishments, not simply individual physicians, are essential to the future of health care. Iltis gives four prudential grounds as to why the government ought to encourage diversity in health care organizations within society. Firstly, private institutions are by their nature diverse and such institutions reduce the burden on the existing government funded system by offering a diversity of health care options. Secondly, diversity along with competition and the potential for profit promotes efficiency, innovation, and technological progress. Thirdly, any system that restricts diversity and requires material equality usually ends up providing uniformly lower levels of care. Lastly, private institutions can limit the overuse that is encouraged by welfare-based health care systems. For all these reasons, health care systems, social policies, and laws should support the diversity and particular integrity of health care institutions.

Iltis underscores the importance of institutional integrity. She points out that only those organizations that have moral commitments can have moral integrity. Integrity is not a binary condition: one does not either have or not have it. Instead, integrity is realized in degrees. However, the integrity of moral commitments is the lens through which we can make moral judgments about individuals and health care organizations. Iltis argues that institutional integrity is the condition for trust in the field of health care, for it allows persons in community to act in their understanding of the human good and of human flourishing. It is also important because of the role of trust in physicians and health care organizations. Individual patients who have moral commitments different from their physicians and health care providers may not trust those physicians and providers. This state of affairs, Iltis argues, can only be solved when health care institutions offer and protect a diversity of understandings of moral integrity. Iltis then turns to how a diversity of health care institutions can and ought to preserve their integrity with the result that there can be a diversity of health care institutions with their own senses of moral integrity. For an organization fully to realize its integrity, it must first have moral commitments and then be at liberty to decide how those commitments will be cashed out in practice. These fundamental commitments must also be understood as normative for the organization as a whole. If these institutions are private they should be permitted to have moral commitments different from the dominant culture, thus allowing the realization in community of particular visions of the human good and human flourishing. Institutional moral diversity not only drives competition and benefits the health care market with a plurality of goods and services, but also takes seriously human moral diversity.

Ruiping Fan offers the last contribution to this section, "A Reconstructionist Confucian Approach to Chinese Health Care: The Ethical Principles, the Market, and Policy Reforms". He argues that, for health care reform in China to be successful, the ethical values and principles of Confucianism must be reconstructed and applied to guide policy. Confucian moral principles must be reclaimed because they, along with Chinese families and other social institutions that were crippled by the Cultural Revolution during the 1960s, are key to China's moral and financial future. They offer social coherence, moral direction, and a view of public policy free of the moral, demographic, political, and virtue hazards. Fan argues further that the two fundamental Confucian moral principles that should guide health care reform in China are the principles of *ren-yi* and the principle of *cheng-xin*. *Ren-yi* translates to humanity-righteousness. Confucius identifies *ren*, a fundamental human virtue, as the quality of "loving humans". Loving other humans is not egalitarian. It begins first and foremost with one's own family. Even though this principle calls for loving all humans, it requires that love should not be given equally to all humans because naturally there will be those humans, such as family members, who have a greater claim to one's love. Confucian love is a love with distinctions. In order to love all humans appropriately, the Confucian must distinguish among people. So in practicing universal human love, love for one's family should nevertheless be emphasized.

The elimination of self-deception is central to the kind of sincerity that *cheng* represents; it is exemplified by a deep commitment to the other Confucian virtue mentioned in this paper, *ren-yi*. *Cheng-xin* can be translated as sincerity-fidelity. *Cheng* is not merely a state of mind or a mental attitude, but a way of being. *Xin* implies that one should be careful about choosing one's words and not using them to deceive others so that one is trustworthy in dealings with others. *Cheng-xin* has the overall implication of maintaining the unity of one's words and deeds, so that in so doing one is being trustworthy in dealing with others. In addition and centrally, Confucian moral principles recognize that the family is the most important component of a society. The family is therefore the most basic social unit for taking care of its own members' welfare. The welfare of its members is a duty of the family. Any support for the weak and the poor should then be family-centered, virtue-sensitive, and essentially non-egalitarian. Welfare in this context is not based on a claim right as to social-welfare entitlement, but instead, it is offered out of sympathy, love, or charity. In this Confucian account, government support should be restricted to those weak groups who do not have a traditional family structure to support them, such as widows, widowers, orphans, the childless, the handicapped, and those harmed by unusual natural disasters. In health care reform in China, the family should therefore be the central locus of health care funding for its members. Through savings and health insurance, the family should bear the burden of the health care costs for its own members out of love and sympathy for those family members. Fan argues that the best implementation of such a system thus far is Singapore's, and that this is the model that China should follow in introducing Confucian moral values in Chinese health care policy.

The next section of this volume opens with "Health Care Services, Markets, and the Confucian Moral Tradition: Establishing a Humanistic Health Care Market" by Zhizheng Du. Du argues that because governments around the world have been unable to provide free health care for all their citizens, market mechanisms have been introduced into the health care system. Since health care, so he contends, is a basic right, medical services should not be bought and sold in the market like other commodities. Yet, the market has proven to be the primary source of innovation and improvement in the level of health care. The result is a fundamental tension. He seeks to mediate this tension by an appeal to traditional Chinese moral principles that, he argues, should be injected into the market so as to create a structure that conforms to a Confucian understanding of human nature. According to the author, the reform of Chinese health care has taken place in four stages. The first stage began in 1987 when the State Council introduced a management system to improve the efficiency of health care services. These reforms made it "so [that] hospitals could be self-managing, responsible for profits and losses, and have self-renewing commodity management" (ms. 1). The second stage of reforms began in 1990. These reforms centered on establishing an administrative system that could meet the demands of a market economy within the basic structure of Chinese health care law. The third stage began in 1997. It recognized that health care is a public concern that should be addressed through market reforms undertaken in the pursuit of efficiency. Policy changes were embraced in order to combine central planning with the power of the market; these changes led to a clearer distinction between for-profit and non-profit hospitals. These reforms also involved expanding the ability of state-run hospitals to make their own decisions locally and to control the prices for their services. There was also the creation of a limited medical insurance program underwritten by personal contributions and government funding. The fourth stage of reforms began in 2004. It seeks to continue the measures of the third stage coupled with providing "better management regulations, convenient healthcare services, and reasonable prices for healthcare services" (ms. 3).

These reforms have had four major effects. Hospitals that introduced market mechanisms are now able to choose what services they will provide, more effectively direct their employees' energies, and more effectively use their own facilities. Secondly, because of the market reforms, healthcare providers are able more successfully to meet the needs of patients. Thirdly, given the better engagement of their healthcare employees, hospitals have been able to expand the number of beds without greatly expanding their number of employees. Lastly, hospital management has been freed to make decision independently of a central bureaucracy allowing hospitals to meet the particular needs of their patients by employing new techniques and technologies. At the same time, these market reforms have had five significant drawbacks. By introducing market elements into healthcare, hospitals have begun to pursue profits along with the health and well-being of their patients. Secondly, the commercialization of health care led to a rapid increase in spending on health care. There is now a market for health care services. Hospitals have also increased the range of their charges and patients have come to make medical decisions on the basis of cost. Market forces have to some extent supported an unequal distribution of health care (which already existed in China) by engaging on larger hospitals in urban areas. Moreover, hospitals no longer focus as much on preventive medicine and primary care, because these services are not as profitable. There is also an inequality in health care because numerous hospitals of various sorts are now able to provide health care. Lastly, the introduction of the profit motive in health care, given the remaining state constraints, has encouraged bribes and kickbacks, given the perverse incentives of the anti-market constraints left from the past (as when bribes provided the only easy avenue to purchase the better care now available, and to reward physicians for their better skills). This last point deserves special emphasis. It was the state's constraint on the ability of patients to pay more for better basic care that drove patients to offer bribes. It was centralized planning that encouraged physicians to offer inappropriate diagnostic and therapeutic interventions in the pursuit of adequate remuneration. These are failures not of the market, but of an appropriate public policy.

According to Du, because of these negative outcomes, regulating healthcare services by market forces alone is not sufficient. Many if not most of the adverse results are a consequence of the failure of appropriate law and public policy, not the market itself. As Du acknowledges, it would be difficult if not impossible to prevent entirely market forces from entering into the medical field. Health care markets must be modified. In providing health care, strengthening health care institutions, and defending the interests of patients, while at the same time making a profit, hospitals must distinguish among those services that should be directed primarily by the market and those that should not. Moreover, trust must remain at the foundation of the physician/patient relationship. Physicians ought to provide those services, which patients need, not merely those services for which patients are able to pay. The challenge will be to fund those services that patients need, but for which they cannot pay. The author suggests that the Confucian notion of kindheartedness should be the guiding principle in healthcare. He proposes it as a remedy to the problems of the commercialization of the medical field.

In the next contribution in this section, "Markets, Trust, and the Nurturing of a Culture of Responsibility: Implications for Health Care Policy in China", Frederic Fransen investigates the constitution of a genuine culture of responsibility in health care. Fransen argues that the core elements of a culture of responsibility are families and communities, along with market relations, which govern the interaction of families within communities and of families and communities with each other. Drawing on the example of the Amish in the United States, Fransen proposes a view of how family-centered cultures such as the Chinese can adapt market reforms in health care. The Amish, living mostly in small farming communities, in their interaction with American society at large are largely unidirectional. That is, they are often generous to outsiders with whom they come into contact, while they are incredibly reluctant to accept aid and support from those outside their communities. This ethos has been the source of conflict with state, local, and federal governments. For example, the Amish do not wish to participate in social security, neither do they purchase insurance (including health insurance). They also do not educate their children beyond the eighth grade.[1] Amish families are large and patriarchal. In addition, as with Confucians, thc family is considered the most basic economic unit, as opposed to the individual. Despite their peculiarity, the Amish fully participate in the market economy around them, within the limits imposed by their religious beliefs.

Fransen argues that, in order for China to foster a culture of responsibility, China must create an institutional framework that allows the family to be the focus of economic decision-making. Moreover, the state must not only protect property from theft and breaches of contract, but it must also create a stable legal environment (i.e., a rule of law) within which families can participate in the market and pass their property from one generation's control to the next. Fransen endorses both Singapore and Hong Kong as models for China to follow, although Singapore is the more interesting model because of the high degree of familial responsibility it underscores and because of its establishment of compulsory savings accounts. Fransen concludes his paper with the recommendation that decisions with regard to the use of health care should be left to appropriate family or community (not societal or governmental) institutions.

The last contribution to this section by Jeremy Garrett, "Fostering Professional Virtue in the Market: Reflections on the Challenges Facing Chinese Health Care Reform", addresses the role of the market in the provision and allocation of health care, as well as the place of private health care institutions. He further argues that "there are good reasons to hold that, in a health care market where (1) health care consumers have good data regarding quality of care and the integrity of health care professionals and (2) where the rule of law is taken seriously, private institutions will nurture, not undermine, the quality of health care." (ms. 1). Garrett further explains why many people have a misplaced antipathy towards markets in health care. First, he suggests that there is a mistake between markets and many adverse health care outcomes that have been experienced in China. For example, many if not most of the untoward outcomes are the result of circumstances that are due to the lack of the necessary pre-requisites for markets to operate properly such as supporting institutions and the rule of law. Secondly, people have a distrust of market forces allocating health care because they view health care as being in some way fundamentally different from other commodities, such that health care has come to be regarded as a right. Lastly, those who oppose the market's role in health care have an inflated confidence in public and/or non-profit health care systems. Despite these common concerns and misperceptions, Garrett claims, "market-based systems for health care delivery are not, in principle, at a qualitative and/or moral disadvantage when compared with their counterparts" (ms. 8). In fact ultimately, virtue has a crucial role to play in ensuring the long-term success of market-based health care systems. Virtue as a strategy helps maximize profits because long-term success in the market depends upon a perception by patients of both reliability and quality, which professional virtue helps to foster (Engelhardt, 1991; Engelhardt & Rie, 1992).

The final section opens with Ren-zong Qiu's "On the Reform of Health Care Reform". According to Qiu, health care reforms in China have had both negative and positive results. While the capacity to diagnose and treat illnesses has dramatically increased in the past third century of health care reforms, 90% of respondents were unsatisfied with the health care reforms. Also, 48.9% of Chinese reported that they had not seen a doctor although they were ill, and 29.6% who could have been admitted to hospitals were not. The data do not show that these were on balance misguided decisions. Even though income has increased 8.9% in urban areas and 2.4% in rural areas from 1995 to 2000, health care costs increased by 13.5% in urban areas and 11.8% in rural over that same period of time. Moreover, health care payouts by the Chinese government decreased from 36.2% of the total to 17.2%. Payments by the society at large have decreased from 42.6 to 27.3%, while individual expenses increased from 21.2% to 55.5% and even up to 60% in 2001. Total health care costs paid by the government in China are only 39.40% of the total health care expenditures (compared with the American situation where 45% of health care was governmentally supported [Levit et al., 2003]). In these circumstances, the central Chinese government is regarded by some Chinese as withdrawing from the field of health care. The central government in provided for only 6.5% of total national health care expenditures in 2000. In 1993, 79.0% of inhabitants in urban areas were covered by medical insurance; in 2003 only 43.0% were. However, from the standpoint of the government, where these health care reforms were intended to lessen the government's economic burden by avoiding the moral and demographic hazards besetting social welfare states, these changes can be regarded as successful. If the difficulties of the welfare state are kept in view, these changes represent a recognition of the moral, demographic, and political hazards of a welfare state and a movement towards a Singaporean solution, insofar as health savings accounts have been established.

Qiu argues then that the market cannot solve all the problems besetting health care in China, but that a system where the state is the sole provider is even worse. As Qiu observes, the market cannot "guarantee social justice, provide non-profit preventive and medical services, provide health care to the vulnerable, and protect the environment, etc." (ms. 8). These are the services, he contends, for which the government should be responsible. He is also of the view that market reforms in health care have distorted the real purpose of hospitals, moving them towards pursuing profits at the expense of caring for patients. However, he raises the possibility of one solution proposed by Engelhardt to health care financing, whereby all would have access to some basic health care, though not the best basic care (Engelhardt, 1996, chap. IV). This will require acknowledging that there will be inequality in the availability of basic health care, and that patients and families will be required to understand and responsibly deal with the cost of health care services they may want to receive. In short, Qiu confronts the central question of the appropriate role of the government in health care.

J. T. Ho provides the final contribution to this volume, "Is Singapore's Health Care System Morally Problematic? A Philosophical Analysis". In Singapore, the health care system compasses both a private and a public health care system. Patients are classified by both their income and their willingness to pay for healthcare. There are six classes of health care services: A1, A2, B1 (air-conditioned), B1 (non-air-conditioned), B2, and C. The first three classes are available in private hospitals where patients pay 100% of their costs. In government hospitals, patients may pay as little as 19% of their total costs, depending on how they are classified. Central to all of this is a mandatory savings plan, Medisave, whereby all employees contribute 20% of their income, and their employers contribute 13% of the employee's salary into an individualized medical savings account. These accounts generate interest at market related rates. There are also two low-cost catastrophic health insurance plans, Medishield and Eldershield, intended to meet the costs of hospitalization when the Medisave account has insufficient funds. There is also a welfare plan, Medifund, established by the government to pay the health care costs of the medically indigent, who are unable to pay for their own medical expenses despite government subsidies.

Ho explores some criticisms of Singapore's system, in particular, those of Michael Barr who has claimed that Singapore's system limits the autonomy of those in the middle and lower classes because their Medisave and Medishield accounts cannot cover certain procedures that people with their own funds can opt to purchase (Barr, 2001). Barr's arguments depend on a claim that people have a moral right to such care and that existing government controls on health care procedures in Singapore deny access to what could be categorized as basic health care. Lastly, Barr criticizes the moral view that poor people should pay for the medical care of their poor relatives. In addressing these criticisms, Ho points out that the first and basic criticism depends on the plausibility of the claim that a positive account of autonomy can create an overriding moral consideration that can justify claim rights to health care. However, Singaporeans with their Confucian heritage find it compelling to rank values, including such autonomy concerns, differently from Westerners such as Barr. Barr's second criticism also depends on the plausibility of the assumption that persons have a claim right to basic health care against the society in which they live, that this right is not trumped by other rights, and that some of those services not subsidized by Singapore's government actually qualify as the basic health care to which one should be entitled by those rights. Barr's third criticism that the ability of family members to use their Medisave accounts to pay for their family members leads to the poor subsidizing the medical treatment of other poor people. This observation as a criticism depends on the view that the poor have a right to have their basic health care needs met through taxation of those who are better off in society. However, the Confucian value placed on the family is a cardinal element of Singapore's culture and morality. If communitarianism is defensible, then to claim that Singapore's system is in this regard unjust does not carry weight. Barr in criticizing the Singapore health care system demonstrates the cleft between the moral assumptions underlying and framing China's Confucian heritage versus those invoked to give legitimacy to the Western European social welfare approach.

3 Looking to China's Future: Taking Confucian Morality, the Rule of Law, and the Market Seriously

The essays in this volume offer a diversity of perspectives on the health care challenges facing contemporary China. China will need to chart a course that can lead it past the disasters that now confront Western welfare states with aging populations, increasing health care costs, and unmet expectations. The West made promises to its people that it cannot fulfill. Even so, the West has been able to postpone its confrontation with reality because it became rich before it became old. China does not have this luxury, because it is becoming old before the majority of its population has become rich. To avoid the catastrophes of the West, the Chinese will need to take seriously their own cultural resources. They will need to draw lessons of success from other Asian polities such as Singapore. China, in framing health care policy, will in particular need to recognize and rightly nourish the inclination to engage in the market and pursue profit, which has created the economic miracle of China since 1978. Among other things, this will mean not blaming or punishing the market for failures of law and governmental policy drawn from a set of ideological commitments that framed Chinese society and economic structure prior to 1978.

In particular, this will involve China's acknowledging that much of the corruption in health care it confronts is predominantly due to bad public policy and law, rather than to the venality of physicians and patients. Physicians are inclined to provide inappropriate drugs and therapies as means of securing financial reward because their remuneration is held artificially low and a system of payment and bonuses is in place that rewards such behaviors. In addition, when patients find that they cannot simply pay for better basic care but are constrained to bribe, and when physicians find that they cannot legally charge for providing better basic care, it is understandable that corruption occurs. Law and public policy established perverse economic rewards and forbade extra pay for better services. The way out of this morass is not to condemn those who were corrupted, but to alter the policy that made corrupt practices reasonable. The establishment of a health care policy that can morally and economically bring China to the future will require a better appreciation of what can be expected from the market, and what must be attributed to seemingly appropriate but nevertheless misdirecting health law and health care policies. China has the opportunity to lead the world to the future. To do this, it will need to face the constraints of human finitude. This is a moral task, requiring a robust moral vision.

Here one confronts the cardinal issue. What resources does China possess for such a moral vision? Given China's cultural past, this question is equivalent to the question of the extent to which Confucian moral resources are available for the task of morally re-invigorating and directing the medical profession, as well as of providing a basis for the moral integrity of families. Drawing on this capital is a formidable but unavoidable challenge. As Ruiping Fan underscores, the response to these challenges will define the China of tomorrow. China needs cultural resources on which it can draw in order to frame a moral vision that is its own. If China is able to escape the demographic hazard, encourage familial responsibility, and avoid the egalitarian moral clichés that have justified the Western social welfare approach to health care and its consequent difficulties, China may yet lead the world not only economically but morally.

Note

[1] In the case of *Wisconsin* vs *Yoder*, 406 U.S. 205 (1972), the United States Supreme Court ruled that the Amish are permitted to withdraw their children from public education once they reach the age of 14, although the legally mandated age was set at 16.

References

Barr, M. (2001). Medical savings accounts in Singapore: A critical inquiry. *Journal of Health Politics, Policy and Law,* 26(4), 709–726.

Engelhardt, H. T., Jr. (1991). Virtue for hire: Some reflections on free choice and the profit motive in the delivery of health care. In T. J. Bole & W. B. Bondeson (Eds.), *Rights to health care* (pp. 327–353). Dordrecht: Kluwer.

Engelhardt, H. T., Jr., & Rie, M. (1992). Selling virtue: Ethics as a profit-maximizing strategy in health care delivery. *Journal of Health & Social Policy, 4*(1), 27–35.

Engelhardt, H. T., Jr. (1996). *The foundations of bioethics* (2nd ed.). New York: Oxford.

Engelhardt, H. T., Jr. (Ed.). (2006). *Global bioethics.* Salem, Massachusetts: M & M Scrivener Press.

Levit, K., Smith, C., Cowan, C., Lazenby, H., Sensenig, A., & Catlin, A. (2003). Trends in U.S. health care spending, 2001. *Health Affairs, 22*(1), 154–164.

Part II
Health Care Policy in China

Towards a Confucian Approach to Health Care Allocation in China: A Dynamic Geography

Yongfu Cao, Yunling Wang, and Linjuan Zheng (Translated by Li Yanwen)

1 Introduction

China began its large scale social and economic reform in 1978, and by 1994, the final aim of the economic restructuring was met. A market economic system was established which had a substantial effect on China's health care system. In the course of the reform, China, introduced and absorbed useful experiences from different countries concerning health care systems. However, China must also provide an emphasis on Chinese culture by giving it an active role in the reform and evolution of its health care system, because Confucianism, the core of traditional Chinese culture, is still influential in every aspect of social life in China.

Confucian philosophy is a human-oriented philosophy that recognizes morality and virtue as the top priority, as the fundamental point for solving issues concerning people's lives and social affairs, and as the basic principle of maintaining the existence of the family, state and society (Zhou & Yan, 2002). According to Renzong Qiu and Xiaomei Zhai (2003), Confucian culture emphasizes that between heaven and earth, human beings are the most valuable existence, because human beings have their internally valuable character and because everyone has dignity as a human being. The basic concept of Confucian ethics is humanity. The benevolent man loves others, and loving people is shown through one's care and respect towards others, and is to take others' attention, benefits, values and viewpoints into one's own consideration. The golden tenet of humanity is that the man of perfect virtue, wishing to be established himself, seeks also to establish others; wishing to be enlarged himself, he seeks also to enlarge others. In addition, another tenet of humanity is not to do to others as you would not wish done to yourself. The Confucian concept of medical treatment as the principle, and humanity as the method, makes a direct connection between Confucianism and bioethics. Xiaoyang Chen and Yongfu Cao (2002) state that the way to humanity is by loving others. Consequently, performing medical practice to provide treatment and save lives is one of the best instruments to lay love upon others. This humanity which saves lives naturally becomes the professional

Y. Cao
Medical Ethics Institute, Medical School, Shandong University, Shandong, China
e-mail: cyongfu@sdu.edu.cn

J. Tao (ed.), *China: Bioethics, Trust, and the Challenge of the Market*,

© Springer Science+Business Media B.V. 2008

standard of the medical community. Evidently, it is of great theoretical importance and practical significance to analyze China's health care system and provide suggestions to certain health care policies by utilizing the concept of people as the foremost, the benevolent man loving others and medical treatment as the principle, and humanity as the method in Confucian philosophy, culture, and ethics.

2 China's Health Care System Before the Social and Economic Restructuring Towards a Market-oriented Reform

2.1 Choices in the Health Care System Before the Economic Restructuring

After the founding of the People's Republic of China in 1949, the health care system that was gradually established consisted of labor-protection health care and free health care in cities and collectively-funded or later called cooperative health care in rural areas.

Labor-protection health care is a scheme adopted in 1951 for employees working in state-run, public-private-joint-run, private-run, and cooperative-run factories, mines and their supporting and affiliated work units. The scope was enlarged to other sectors such as railways, shipping, post and telecommunications, road transportation, architecture and so on. The major protection measures are as follows: (1) Employees injured at work could enjoy paid medical leave and free diagnosis, treatment, medicine, hospitalization, meals during hospitalization and transportation to the hospital, which were all borne by the enterprise they worked for; (2) Ill or not-on-the-work injured employees, in visiting appointed hospitals, could enjoy free diagnosis, treatment, surgery, hospitalization and ordinary medicine, which were all borne by the enterprise; (3) Costs on expensive or exceptional medicines, meals during hospitalization and transportation to the hospital were to be paid by the patient themselves; (4) The employees could reimburse half of the medical expenses in the appointed hospitals on diagnosis, treatment, surgery and ordinary medicines from their enterprises for the linear relative under their support but needed to pay other costs by themselves.

The free health care scheme was a system to give free medical care to those working for government offices or public institutions, as well as university students. From July 1952 on, the free health care system was enlarged in stages to governments at various levels, different parties, political organizations such as the trade union, the youth league and the women's association, various working teams, public institutions such as cultural, educational, health, and economic undertakings, and revolutionary disabled service men. Extension was made to include university students, poly-technical college students and cadres at the township-level into this system in 1953. Further, a decision was made on June 29, 1956, that retired government officials and workers would still be entitled to free health care.

Cooperative health care service in rural areas, oriented to serve all the members living in the community and based on their mutual cooperation, was a health care scheme with Chinese characteristics that helped raise funds through individual contributions combined with governmental or collective subsidies, and gave reimbursement in certain proportions to community members for their medical treatment and prevention expenses. Initiated by people at the grass-roots level in the 1950s, the system experienced great development later owing to the positive assessment of Mao Zedong in 1966. "By 1980, about 90% of the administrative villages (production brigades) in China had implemented the system of cooperative health care service. 'Cooperative health care service', the relevant 'health stations', and numerous 'bare-foot doctors' are the three 'magic weapons' in solving the problem of shortage of doctors and medicine in rural areas" (Qiao, 2004).

2.2 Evaluation Upon the Old Health Care System

2.2.1 The Old Health Care System was Established to be Geared to the Planned Economy

Free health care and labor-protection health care were the outcome of planned economy. At that time, the state took planned measures to exercise highly centralized management over medical resources, and exerted unitary administration over the production, distribution, exchanges and consumption of the medical resources, resulting in unified planning for all these functions, and concentrated integration of the ownership, operation and use of the medical resources.

The consolidation and development of cooperative health care in rural areas also took place during the time of planned economy. Collective rural economic organizations, funded by collective economic resources and regarded highly, and thus supported by governments at various levels, provided support for the development of cooperative health care.

2.2.2 The Old Health Care System Embodied Great Ethical Value

The health care system of new China embodied the ethical vision of "serving the people's health," as well as representing the Confucian concepts of "people as the foremost; the benevolent man loving others; and medical treatment as the principle and humanity as the method." At that time, all the social undertakings were based on people's fundamental interests, the medical cause being no exception. The National Conference on Public Health Work convened by the Ministry of Public Health in Beijing in August 1950, set up three principles in the work of public health, one of which was that medical work should "serve workers, farmers and soldiers", i.e. the medical system established by the new government cared about people's health, embodied social fairness and consequently represented great ethical value.

The old health care system, under that historical circumstance, played an active role in promoting the development of the health care cause, protecting employees' health, enhancing economic construction and safeguarding social security. "When the new government was established in 1949, the health indexes of the Chinese people were categorized to the lowest country group. By the end of the 1970s, China had become one of the countries with the most complete health care system, with 80–85% of the population enjoying basic health care. All this was attributed to three kinds of health care systems implemented since the 1950s (Li & Wang, 2004, p. 9).

The most praiseworthy among the three was cooperative health care service in the rural areas. China is a big country of agriculture and the provision of health care to farmers is pertinent to the overall level of health care in the whole country. On June 26, 1965, Mao Zedong instructed that "Emphasis of medical work should be given to rural areas." This was very effective in promoting rural medical work and rural cooperative health care service. "The mode of cooperative health care service was praised by the WHO and World Bank as 'the only example to solve the problem of health expenditure in developing countries' and was promoted as a model among the third world countries" (Song, 2004, p. 24).

2.2.3 Limitation of the Old Health Care System

The old health care system was established under a planned "supply-oriented" economy with comparatively low-level productivity. Consequently, the health care services that people enjoyed were very limited in both urban and rural areas. Because of the progress of economic reform, the disadvantages of the traditional health care system became more apparent.

The major demerits of free health care and labor-protection health care include the following:

(1) Because the state and various enterprises covered almost all the medical expenses for urban employees, the employees paid very little towards their health care costs and they became very indifferent and unaware of the actual expenditures. As a result, people frequently utilized the health care services offered. Often people sought expensive treatments for minor ailments or tried to get medical treatments for their whole family. Unavoidably, the medical expenditure increased very fast and incurred a huge waste on medical resources. Since the advent of social and economic reform, the total income volume of the employees all over China increased from RMB 56.89 billion in 1978, to RMB 929.65 billion in 1998, an increase of 16.34 times, while the increase of free health care and labor-protection health care was far more higher than that of the income: RMB 3.16 billion in 1978, and RMB 77.37 billion in 1997, an increase of 24.48 times (Cai, 2000).
(2) The old health care system operated at a very low level of management and socialization. There was a large difference in the health care service offered to employees working in different places. In addition, quite a number of people could not get basic health care service.
(3) The health care system only covered a limited number of people working in public owned enterprises, state organizations and public institutions. However,

with the progress in economic restructuring, a large number of non-public owned enterprises emerged, such as individual enterprises, private enterprises, and foreign-involved enterprises. Employees in these enterprises could not enjoy basic health care. Apart from that, numerous unemployed urban dwellers were also excluded from the medical system (Hu & Leng, 2004).

The major demerits of cooperative medical service in rural areas include the following:

(1) The lack in legal control over the implementation of the stipulation of cooperative health care resulted in delayed or no contribution to the fund-raising, or delayed or no reimbursement to the medical expenses owing to deficit in the medical budget.
(2) The fund for cooperative health care was mainly shared by collectives and individuals and the rate of reimbursement was decided by different towns and villages. There was often no standard or authorized organization to make prudent investigation, scientific analysis and precise calculation to give a reasonable basis for assessment.
(3) Since the cooperative health care service was provided by individual towns and villages, the source of funds relied mainly on collective economic organizations and individual farmers. This led to limited contributions, lesser margin for more funds, and greater vulnerability to risks.
(4) The cooperative health care system often changed with the change of mind of the leader in charge or the change of the administrative group. The cooperative health care system lacked stability. For example, it might be in force in spring, but later stopped in autumn or be supported this year and abandoned the next (Liang, 2003, p. 98).

In a word, the original health care system became increasingly unfit for the new economic system. Labor-protection health care "diverted enterprises' financial and human resources and affected production and business operation. In enterprises with poor economic returns, the employees could not be cared by the basic health care service" (Liang, 2003). After the implementation of the household-contract responsibility system in rural areas, the cooperative health care system collapsed immediately. "A study carried out in 1985 showed that after the disappearance of the people's commune, the number of administrative villages still adopting cooperative health care dropped sharply from 90% to 5%. The figure dropped further to 4.8% in 1989" (Wang, 2003).

3 Reform of the Health Care System in China

To be in pace with the market economy, the reform of the health care system in China started from the establishment of basic health care and increasingly touched upon other supporting protection systems. This paper hereby makes an introduction to and a comment on the basic health care insurance system in urban areas, the cooperative health care system in rural areas and the commercial medical insurance system.

3.1 The Ethical Principles of the Reform in China's Health Care System

In the process of health care reform, China has attached great importance to the mission of ethical values. According to our *Constitution*, "Citizens of the People's Republic of China have the right to material assistance from the state and society when they are old, ill or disabled. The state develops the social insurance, social relief and medical and health services that are required to enable citizens to enjoy this right." Article 98 of the *General Code of Civil Law* also stipulates: "Citizens are entitled with the right to life and health." To define the citizens' entitlement to health as a basic right and as one of the obligations that government should do its utmost to fulfill the clarified government's duty in building a social health care system and in providing ethical backup and legal assurance for the establishment and development of the medical system.

In the guiding document for national health and medical care reform, *Resolutions on Health Reform and Development*, the following provisions can be found: "We should stick to the principle of serving the people, correctly handle the relationship between social benefits and economic returns, giving first priority to social benefits. The tendency to seek economic returns and neglect social benefits must be guarded against." "Focusing on the improvement of people's health, priority should be given to the development and assurance of basic health service to embody social fairness and gradually satisfy people's diversified requirement."

In order to explore the ethical principle for medical reform, the Bioethical Branch of China Federation of Medicine convened a national symposium to discuss the ethical principles that medical reform should follow. The symposium decided that health and medical reform must abide by the following principles: (1) public good first; (2) broad coverage; (3) all-round beneficiaries; (4) fair distribution; (5) high quality service; (6) health responsibility; (7) free choice; and (8) public participation. This is of great constructive importance to medical and health care reform.

However, we must realize that there is an insufficient emphasis on traditional culture, especially Confucian ethics in the course of medical care reform. In particular there is a lack of focus on benevolence, medical treatment as the principle, humanity as the method, and valuing justice above material gains (Zhao & Song, 1999).

3.2 Reform of Urban Medical Insurance and Its Ethical Evaluation

In 1998, the State Council decided to reform the basic medical insurance system for employees in cities and towns. This reform, based on the capacity of the government budget, enterprises, and individuals, was intended to establish a system that can meet the requirement of the market economy and fill employees' basic medical needs.

The basic urban medical insurance scheme included the following features: (1) The basic medical insurance premium should be shared by both the employer and the employee in rational proportions; (2) The basic medical insurance fund is composed of combined contributions from various sources in society with personal accounts; (3) The contributions from various sources in society and personal accounts, separated and irreplaceable from each other, cover different payments; (4) The scheme is to be carried out at various levels with the prefecture as the basic unit for social contributions, and all the employers and employees should take part in the scheme in conformity with the regulations of the administrative region; (5) Public institutions managing the social insurance should shoulder the responsibility for raising, controlling and the payment of the basic medical insurance fund, institutionalize their work and accept the supervision of relevant state and public organizations; (6) Effective management mechanisms should be established for medical insurance services.

The urban health care insurance scheme in China has absorbed the internationally practiced mode of social insurance and medical savings accounts. As the major scheme of the urban health care system, it has, to some extent, made up for the dysfunction of the market mechanism, represented the obligations of the society for public health, and showed social fairness. At present, this scheme attempts to cover people of all professions and income levels in cities and towns, including the retired, and will by and large cover all those who can afford the insurance premiums for themselves and their family members.

The new medical insurance scheme has changed the situation of the state and enterprises taking on all the medical responsibility and thus reducing their heavy medical expenditure; it makes clear the rational rate of the medical expenses shared between the state, enterprises and individuals, restrained unjustified demand for health care by individuals, and enhanced people's consciousness of rights, benefits and obligations. However, problems still exist, such as "improper management of the personal accounts in the basic medical insurance plans, difficulty in being included in the scheme for employees working in enterprises running at a loss, overhigh medical expenses for some patients, the coverage of the scheme remaining to be extended, and so on" (Xu, 2004).

3.3 Rural Cooperative Health Care Scheme and Its Ethic Evaluation

China is a big agricultural country with 60% of its population living in rural areas. Solving farmers' health care problems is pertinent to a successful reform of China's health and medical reform. "At the beginning of the 1990s, the Chinese government made a mission statement to the WHO that China would commit to making an overall improvement on the basic-level health and medical work in rural areas by the year 2000. In line with that goal, the government put forward the program of 'restoring and regenerating' the cooperative health care service. But for many reasons, the mission did not proceed smoothly and ended in failure in most pilot regions" (Wang, 2003). In spite of more than ten years' effort, the rural cooperative health care system has not been rebuilt as expected, and people covered by the service has always been less than 10%. According to "The Third National Survey on Health Service" conducted by the Ministry of Public Health in 2003, only 8.8% of the population in China enjoys cooperative health care.

For this reason, the Ministry of Public Health, Ministry of Finance, and Ministry of Agriculture jointly promulgated "Opinions on the Establishment of New Cooperative Health Care System in Rural Areas", and made the following instructions on the reform of the rural cooperative health care scheme in China in the new period: (1) In the new rural cooperative health care scheme, individual counties (county-level cities) will be the basic units for the medical fund raising from various sources in society, a combination of personal payments, collective support and government subsidies; (2) In accordance with the principle of payment according to income, balance between payments and income, and fairness, openness and impartialness, the earmarked medical fund is saved in a special account and not allowed to be diverted or appropriated for other purposes; (3) Based on the actual situation of different regions, medical establishments in rural areas are designated on a selective basis to provide health care services for farmers, and they will be under strengthened control, supervision and dynamic management.

The new cooperative medical service was a preliminary health care system for farmers, which aimed to provide mutual relief and mutual help for medical treatment and medical prevention. It is based on a collective economy and a collective capability and is organized voluntarily by farmers. The system includes both social welfare and social insurance.

In actual application and promotion of this scheme, there have emerged many problems and difficulties, including insufficient understanding of its benefits, difficulty in fundraising, obscurity in policy, sub-standardization in management and low-level financial sources from the society and so on (Wu, X., 2004).

3.4 Commercial Health Care Insurance and Its Ethical Evaluation

The basic health care schemes are to provide fundamental health and medical services to employees in cities and towns and farmers in rural areas. If demand for health care goes beyond the basic medical scheme, or special needs require service beyond the basic medical demand, then these situations would be solved through the market by commercial medical insurance.

Commercial health care insurance is an insurance plan where the insurer provides reimbursement to the insurant on the medical expenses incurred from accidents or diseases. The market for commercial health care, though still in its initial stage, has functioned positively in the construction of the medical system of the country. For instance, many of the commercial insurance schemes, such as hospitalization medical insurance, serious diseases insurance, various diseases insurance, and students' health insurance, have served as supplementation or substitution to the social health care system. In the meantime, for those who have already taken part in the social health care system but demand higher and better health care service, commercial medical insurance, as a supplementary factor, can provide them with more choices of higher-level health care services. China is a country with a large population and enjoys great market potential for commercial medical insurance. It is quite necessary and helpful to make commercial medical insurance a supplementation to the above-mentioned health care system.

4 Outlook of the Health Care System in China and Obstacles Ahead

4.1 Considerations Upon the Reform of Health Care System in China

At present, the outlook of the reform of the health care system in China is quite clear. In urban areas, a multi-layered health care system will be established with social medical assistance as the foundation, social health care insurance as the main body, the national health service system proving health care service to certain groups of people as part of social welfare, and commercial health care insurance, medical allowances by the employers and various health welfare schemes as supplementations (Wu, R., 2004). In rural areas, the cooperative health care system should be rebuilt, as illustrated by the following Fig. 1:

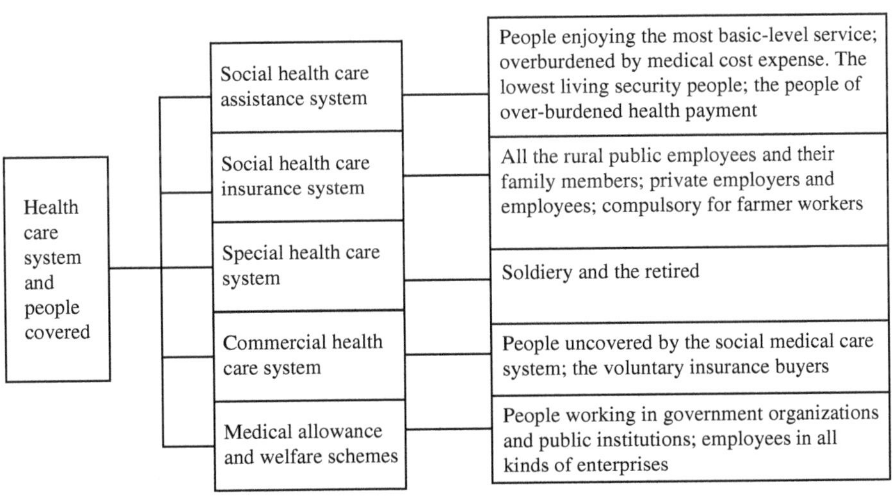

Fig. 1 Cooperative health care system

4.2 Deficiencies and Difficulties in the Development of a Health Care System in China

Despite the clear outlook, there are still some deficiencies and difficulties in the development of a health care system in China as follows:

4.2.1 Narrow Coverage of the Social Health Care Insurance

From the Table 1, it can be seen that the coverage rate of basic health care and cooperative health care is only 44.8% and 79.0% of urban and rural people, respectively, who have to pay the expenses themselves. This means a vast majority of Chinese people do not have institutionalized health care.

4.2.2 Multi-layered Health Care System Yet to be Established

Though China's health care reform is seen in its clear outlook and framework, effective implementation measures must be taken in various institutions for employees' basic health care insurance, employees' supplementary health care insurance, commercial health care insurance, social health care assistance, and rural cooperative health care, etc.

4.2.3 Insufficient Input by the Government

From the above Table 2 it can be seen that though the health expenditure in total has been increasing over the years, government health expenditure has been decreasing, i.e. the public health care expenditure has been decreasing. The insufficient input by the government has affected the health care level of its citizens.

Table 1 Health care insurance system in 2003 (%)

	Total	Urban	Rural
Cooperative Insurance	8.8	6.6	9.5
Basic Insurance	8.9	30.4	1.5
Serious disease Insurance	0.6	1.8	0.1
Government	1.2	4.0	0.2
Labor Insurance	1.3	4.6	0.1
Others	1.4	2.2	1.2
Commercial Insurance	7.6	5.6	8.3
Self payment	70.3	44.8	79.0

Source: *Chinese National Survey on Health Service*, 2003.

Table 2 Health expenditures

	1980	1990	1995	2000	2001	2002
Total Health Expenditure (100 million yuan)	143.2	747.4	2, 155.1	4, 586.6	5, 025.9	5, 684.6
% of Health Expenditures	100.0	100.0	100.0	100.0	100.0	100.0
Government Health Expenditure	36.2	25.1	18.0	15.5	15.9	15.2
Social Health Expenditure	42.6	39.2	35.6	25.5	24.1	26.5
Personal Health Expenditure	21.2	35.7	46.4	59.0	60.0	58.3

Source: *Summary of Chinese statistics on Health Service in* 2004.

4.3 Solution to the Difficulties in China's Health Care Reform

With regard to the above analysis, the writer of this paper argues that importance should be attached to traditional Confucian cultural resources to guide and influence the reform and development of China's health care service and to ensure that government policies and the health care system best embody Confucian ethic concepts of "people as the foremost", "the benevolent man loving others", "medical treatment as the principle and humanity as the method", and "valuing justice above material gains". For this purpose, emphasis should be given to the following:

4.3.1 Government's Obligations

Government plays a leading role in the establishment and reform of a health care system. On the one hand, government should be responsible in drafting and coordinating the implementation of polices, and on the other hand, government should provide financial support for the development and improvement of the system. As a signatory member to "Alma-Ata Declaration", our government should represent the concept of Confucian culture in its policies and bear the responsibility to provide basic health care to each citizen. The government should, with the prerequisite of no increase in taxation, optimize the distribution of public expenditures and increase the financial input to health care. Government's further financial input should mainly be given to these two areas: (1) health care service providers (hospitals), and (2) other health care schemes such as the health care assistance to the weak and poor and the new cooperative health care. This financial input is the foundation for the health care system to run efficiently.

4.3.2 Legal Assurance

A health care system involves the obligations and behaviors of the demanders, suppliers, and the insurance institutions, and requires standardization and regulation of legal institutions. For instance, efforts must be made to strengthen the control over hospitals, to make strict evaluation in designating hospitals and drugstores for the health care system. Meanwhile, individuals should also be educated to be cost-conscious in order to prevent extravagance and health care insurance overspending, and to prevent false claims or fraudulent use of the health care insurance reimbursement, in particular. In addition, the hand-over of insurance funds should also be protected by law in order to ensure the sustained and stable use of the health care insurance fund.

4.3.3 Social Participation

The development and improvement of the health care system, which concerns the benefits of all the households and the health of every citizen, should have the participation of all the social forces and all the citizens so as to promote the perfection of the system. Employers and individuals should actively pay the premiums, and try their best to make insurance coverage bigger. Medical establishments should provide high quality and efficient service. In addition, health care insurance institutions should open the protective umbrella of life by providing timely reimbursement to the insurants in case of diseases or accidents.

References

Cai, R. (2000). Health care insurance and hospital reform. *China Hospital Management, 20*(12), 68.

Chen, X., & Cao, Y. (2002). *Bioethics* (p. 41). Jinan: Shandong University Press.

Hu, Y., & Leng, M. (2004). Transformation of social economy and reform in health care system. *Health Soft Science, 18*(3), 102–103.

Liang, W. (2003). *Health care service management*. Beijing: People's Medical Press.

Li, W., & Wang, J. (2004). Ideas for China's social health insurance system reform. *Modern Finance, 24*(10), 9.

Qiao, Y. (2004). History of China's rural cooperative health care service. *Qinghai Social Science, 25*(3), 66.

Qiu, R., & Zhai, X. (2003). *Introduction to bioethics* (pp. 27–28). China: Peking Union Medical College Press.

Song, B. (2004). The past, present and future of China's rural cooperative health care service. *Medicine and Philosophy, 25*(3), 24.

Wang, S. (2003). *Comparison: Crisis and improvement of China's public health*. Beijing: Zhongxin Press.

Wu, R. (2004). Ideas on China's health care system reform. *International Medicine and Health Guide, 10* (9), 33–34.

Wu, X. (2004). Exploration on rural cooperative health care service Reform. *Zhejiang Preventive Medicine, 16*(12), 64.

Xu, D. (2004). Historical exploration and re-establishment of China's health care system. *Exploration, 24* (5), 115.

Zhao, M., & Song, W. (1999). Facing the new century: Health care reform and medical ethnics – summarization of the 10th national medical ethnics symposium. *Medicine and Philosophy, 20*(11), 24.

Zhou, L., & Yan, B. (2002). *Confucian culture and modern society* (p. 6). Jinan: Shandong University Press.

Trust is the Core of the Doctor–Patient Relationship: From the Perspective of Traditional Chinese Medical Ethics

Benfu Li and Linying Hu

1 Introduction

The traditional doctor–patient relationship is the interpersonal relationship between doctor and patient based on supply and demand. With the development of society and medicine, and the socialization of medicine, this relationship has evolved into the interpersonal relationships between doctor-centered and patient-centered groups. China is experiencing the transition towards a market-oriented system. However, the health care market is far from mature in the absence of an effective management system and self-regulation. In this context, the doctor–patient relationship is confronted with serious challenges from the commercialization of health care. At present, there is an increase in the number of doctor–patient conflicts and dissensions. As a result, the level of doctor–patient trust that has been established and maintained for many years is on the edge of collapse. In my viewpoint, besides health care system reform and morality transformation in accordance with the development of China's market economy, we should advocate traditional medical ethics to rebuild doctor–patient trust. From the perspective of traditional Chinese medical ethics, trust has always constituted the core of doctor–patient relationships. The research on the culture, background, groundwork and conditions of the doctor–patient trust will be very helpful for us to understand the possibilities for trust in doctor–patient relationships in modern health care.

2 The Traditional Moral Cultural Background of Doctor–Patient Trust

Confucianist moral culture was the core of Chinese traditional culture, which attached much importance to trust ("Cheng xin"). In Chinese traditional culture, trust was endued with rich meanings, including integrity, honesty and trustworthi-

B. Li
Department of Medical Ethics, Health Science Center, Peking University
e-mail: libenfubest@126.com

J. Tao (ed.), *China: Bioethics, Trust, and the Challenge of the Market*,
© Springer Science+Business Media B.V. 2008

ness, etc. Confucius said: "I know not what a man without trustworthiness may accomplish. Be it large or small, how could a carriage move without its yoke-bar?" (Confucius, 2005, 2:22). He held that "trust" is a basic moral principle for a person settling down and going on with his pursuits in society. Meanwhile, Confucius also emphasized that policymaking should be trusted by the people first, then the policies could be implemented. Mencius said, "Friends should be trustworthy and trust each other." He listed the "trust" between friends as one of the five basic requirements for interpersonal relationships (Mencius, 2003, T'ang Wan Kung, Part I, 3:4).

Previously "Cheng" and "Xin" were used separately in the ancient language, and in modern times, Chinese people began to use "Cheng xin" jointly. However, if we consider it carefully, we find that there are some subtle differences between them. "Cheng" refers to the unilateral requirements to individual moral agents. "Xin" focuses more on the bilateral or multilateral requirement to social groups. "Cheng" means a certain internal virtue of the moral agent. "Xin" means the internalization of "Cheng" and is presented as socialized moral actions. "Cheng xin" implies that a person is trusted by others in light of his own internal virtue of integrity.

As the part of social interpersonal relationships, the doctor–patient relationship is greatly influenced by the conception of "Cheng xin". Both physicians and patients acknowledge that the trust should be the core of the doctor–patient relationship.

3 The Groundwork of Doctor–Patient Trust

From the perspective of traditional Chinese medical ethics, medicine is a humanitarian career ever since its birth. Liu An of the Han Dynasty said, "Shennong tried the character of all kinds of herbs and waters, so as to make it clear to the public which to choose and which to discard. In doing this, he once encountered more than seventy kinds of poisonous herbs in a single day. And he combined the therapeutical herbs into a recipe to cure people" (Liu, 2004). This ancient Chinese legend has shown that medicine is a humanitarian cause ever since its birth, and this is based on people's confirmation about life sanctity. As Suwen of *Yellow Emperor's Classic of Internal Medicine (Huangtineijing)* said, "Covered by the heaven and carried by the earth is a complete array of all kind of things, of which human beings are the most valuable" (Veith, 2002). Medicine and the doctor's behavior can also significantly affect a person's life. As Zhang Bingcheng of Qing Dynasty said, "medicine bears the rule of nature, and is in charge of life and death" (*Set Recipes of Practical Value*, Author's Preface). So our ancient philosophers and physicians deemed medicine as a benevolent cause, the benevolent love of people, and especially an emphasis on the "love of all the people". At the same time, they saw medical practice as an approach and instrument of loving people. *The Yellow Emperor's Classic of Internal Medicine* stated, "...from the larger view, it can govern the people, from a smaller view, it can cure the people, thus making people healthy and peaceful. The virtue will come down and benefit the future generation..." (Veith, 2002). Moreover, the doctors extended the meanings of "love of all the people" to the equal treatment of all patients. Sun Simiao of the Tang Dynasty said: "We should treat all patients equally as our close kin and good friend, and give them elaborate care, regardless of their wealth, age, appearance, nationality, intellect and relationship with the doctor" (Sun, 2002). In summary, "medicine as benevolence cause" has been the basic principle of traditional Chinese medical ethics, which is shared by doctors in all dynasties. In the course of treating the patient, they will try their best even with very little hope, carelessness about their own personal safety, and sometimes will even give up their own life.

The patients are always put into an inferior position because of the asymmetry of medical knowledge and ability between doctors and patients. Therefore, traditional Chinese medical ethics demands first that the medical practitioner respect the patients and protect the patients' interests. For example, from the Song Dynasty, "Discourse of the Medical Practitioner" in *Method for the Treatment of Children's Diseases* states,[1] "To be a doctor, people should be gentle in character, courteous in treating the patient, seemly in behavior, sedate in action, with no false pride and airs and graces." Gong Tingxian of the Ming Dynasty said, "The patients, once they resort to a doctor, have recommended their life to them, so we should respect them and never despise them. . . " (Gong, 1998). Chen Shigong, who also lived in the Ming Dynasty, said "On treating the women, the doctor must be accompanied, an examination without an attender is not allowed. Diseases difficult to tell especially demand earnest treatment. Moreover, the doctor must keep the secret even from their wives because they are the private affairs of the woman" (Chen, 2002). To summarize, the aforementioned has shown the trustworthiness of doctors and medical practitioners. Meanwhile, the patient's inferior position also disposes them to the requirement that they respect physicians and "not conceal their disease in fear of the medical treatment." For example, Kou Zongshi from the Song Dynasty said, "The patient should not suspect or despise the doctor, or it will bring about disasters" (Kou Zongshi). Also there is Wang Guan of the Ming Dynasty who said: "If the patient conceals the state of his illness, refuses to a therapy, or even be overbearing and indulging with no reason or self-control, they are hard to cure" (Wang, 1995). Under this requirement, most of the patients are open to the doctors, telling their secrets, even defects and crimes. This reflects the high level of trust between patients and their doctors. Meanwhile, it demonstrates that as a profession, medicine can not achieve its own value and not reach its goal without the mutual trust between doctors and patients.

To generalize, traditional Chinese medical ethics endues medicine with ethical values. This and the asymmetry of medical knowledge and ability between doctor and patient constitute the groundwork of doctor–patient trust. At present, although there is a decline in doctor–patient trust, the groundwork of which has not changed. However, this by no means implies we should turn a deaf ear to the present situation. Therefore, we ought to enhance our understanding of medicine's ethics respecting the self-determination of both the doctor and the patient.

4 The Conditions for Doctor–Patient Trust

In order to achieve mutual trust between doctors and patients, traditional Chinese medical ethics put more professional duties and obligations on the side of the medical practitioner. For example, it was written by Sun Simiao that "The value of life is higher than a thousand gold, and if one prescription can help, it values more" (Sun, 2002). Kou Zhongshi in Song Dynasty also wrote that "To make a prescription is like executing penalty; penalty should not be misused, otherwise it will kill undeserved person, so does the use of herb" (Kou Zongshi).

Besides this, traditional medical ethics emphasized a high moral level as the prerequisite for practicing medicine, and formed a complete system of moral cultivation of the medical practitioner. As emphasized in Discourse about Medicine of Self-Communion Notes (Xingxinlu, Yilun) by Lin Fu of Song Dynasty, "One who has no lasting morality can not be a physician, since it concerns human lives." Moral cultivation is prioratized in traditional medical ethics. First, traditional medical ethics emphasized "self-cultivation" and "restraint of the desire for private interests", such as *Discourse of the Medical practitioner of Method of the Treatment of Children's Diseases* of Song Dynasty which states that "the general approach for being a great physician lies in cultivating oneself first before treating patients." The core of self-cultivation is to restrain the desires for private interests. In his Ten Criterions for Physicians in Healing All the Diseases, Gong Tingxian of Ming Dynasty pointed out: "Never pay much attention to profit, just holding a benevolent heart" and made it as the tenth criterion for a good physicians (Gong, 1998). In the author's preface of *A New Book of Pediatric of Song Dynasty*, Liu Fang firmly believed that "a medical practitioner must have a heart of saving people, and mustn't have a heart of selfness" (Liu, 1981). Tang Dynasty famous physician, Sun Simiao, also emphasized that "when a great physician is treating the patient, he needs to first calm himself to the state of no desire or demand. Then he can arouse a heart of great mercy and pity, swear to relieve all the suffered" (Sun, 2002). Second, the cultivation of moral sentiments is the crucial factor for being a good physician. Yu Chang wrote in *Principle and Prohibition for Medical Profession* of Qing Dynasty that "Medicine requires benevolence. A man of honor must possess zealous emotion. Possessing zealous emotion, he then can treat the patient as himself and be detailed when questioning the state of an illness" (Yu, 1983). In *The Scholars*, Wu Jingzhi even held that "A physician should have the spirit of cutting off the flesh in his thigh to save the patient if needed" (Wu, 1992). Third, traditional medical ethics not only attached importance to the cultivation of the moral agent's internal moral commands and moral sentiments, but also developed a complete set of medical professional standards and behavioral norms, which together constitute the important conditions for establishing and maintaining doctor–patient trust, such as "Ten Criterions for Physicians in Healing All the Disease" by Gong Tingxian (Gong, 1998); "Five Prohibitions and Ten Criterions for Physicians" in *Orthodox Manual of External Disease*, by Chen Shigong (Chen, 2002); "Ten Prohibitions for Physicians" in *Zhang's Treatise on General Medicine* by Zhang Shiwan of the Qing Dynasty (Zhang, 1995) and rules of the medical practitioner suggested by Song Guobin in "Medical Ethics during the reign of The Republic of China" (Song, 1933). Correspondingly, physicians also set some rules of conduct for the patient, such as "Admonition for Patients in the Annuals of Ancient and Current Medicine" and "Ten Criterions for Patients in Healing All the Diseases" by Gong Tingxian

(Gong, 1998). These concrete behavior norms for physicians and patients provided the general public rich information on medical practices and ensured doctor–patient trust.

The trend of the commercialization of health care has affected medical professionals. A profit-seeking ethos emerging from the new market economy has eclipsed medical ethics and undermined standards of professional conduct. Unfortunately, we have no effective regulations and professionalism to counteract the negative effects of the commercialization of health care. Thus, it is not rare that doctors request and receive "red envelopes" from patients, receive "kick-backs" from pharmaceutical companies and prescribe the "big prescriptions", etc., which have seriously damaged the patient's interests, increased the conflicts and dissensions between doctors and patients, and have resulted in the crisis of the doctor–patient trust. We should call for traditional Chinese medical ethics to inculpate the spirit of probity, selflessness and dedication, and put the patient's interests first, which may help to improve the tensional status between the doctor and the patient and to rebuild doctor–patient trust. However, it should be noted that the rebuilding of doctor–patient trust is not an isolated process. It should be set within the background of health care system reform. Meanwhile, health care policy-making should consider providing a good institutional background for the cultivation of doctor–patient trust and consolidate the foundation of the trust as well.

Note

[1] The author of *Method for the Treatment of Children's Diseases* (Xiao er wei sheng zong wei fang lun) is unknown. It was published in 1156, Song Dynasty.

References

Chen, S. (2002). Chapter 4. *Orthodox manual of external diseases*. Beijing: Chinese Traditional Medicine.

Confucius. (2005). Chapter 2. In J. Sun & L. Yang (Trans.), *Lunyu*. Changchun: Jilin People Press.

Gong, T. (1998). Chapter 29. *Healing all the diseases*. Beijing: Chinese Traditional Medicine Press.

Kou, Z. (Song Dynasty). *Amplified materia medica,* Author's preface, (Hand-written copy of Qing Dynasty).

Liu, A. (2004). Chapter 19. In J. Wang (Trans.), *Huannanzi*. Guangzhou: Guangzhou Press.

Liu, F. (1981). *A new book of pediatric*, Author's preface. Beijing: Chinese Traditional Medicine Ancient Books Press.

Mencius. (2003). T'ang Wan Kung. In X. Bai (Trans.), *Mencius* (Part I, 3:4). Beijing: People Education Press.

Song, G. (1933). Chapter 1. *Medical ethics*. Shanghai: Guoguang Publishing House.

Sun, S. (2002). Chapter 1. *Prescriptions worth a thousand gold for emergencies*. Beijing: Hualing Press.

Veith, I. (Trans.). (2002). *The yellow emperor's classic of internal medicine*. Berkeley: University of California Press.

Wang, G. (1995). Collection of experiences of famous physicians in the Ming Dynasty. In S. Fengge (Trans.), *Discourse of medicine* (Chapter 1). Beijing: People Health Press.
Wu, C.T. (1992). *The Scholars*. In G. Yang & Y. Hsien-yi (Trans.). New York: Columbia University Press.
Yu, C. (1983). Discourse of asking diseases. In *Principle and prohibition for medical profession* (Chapter 1). Shanghai: Shanghai Science and Technology Press.
Zhang, S. (1995). Preface. In J. Li (Trans.), *Zhang's treatise on general medicine*. Beijing: Chinese Traditional Medicine Press.

Medical Resources, the Market, and the Development of Private-Run Hospitals in China

Xiaoyang Chen, Tongwei Yang, and Xiuqin Shen (Translated by: Yanwen Li)

1 The Present Picture of Utilization of Medical Resources in China

A basic fact in economics is that resources are scarce compared to human demand. Therefore, throughout history the challenge has been to balance limited resources and human beings' limitless desire to consume these resources. Furthermore, these conflicting values result in the basic issue in economics as to how to make use of the limited and scarce resources to produce and provide products in order to maximally satisfy people's infinite demands and desires, and to maximize social welfare. These conflicting values drive economic activity, i.e. rational distribution and efficient use of limited resources and provision of products.

And what is the present situation in China relating to the use of the scarce resources in the field of public health? Since the adoption of reform and an opening-up policy, China's medical enterprises have experienced considerable increases in development, in terms of either the scale of the hospitals and medical organizations, or the quantity and quality of man power, or material supply and financial capacity. Nevertheless, according to our interviews and based on national investigation data in health service, much is to be desired in the utilization of medical resources, owing to specific facts as follows:

1. The overall efficiency of the health service system is to be increased.

Table 1 was created using the "Statistical Summary of China's Health Service" in 2004.

It can be generalized from Table 1 that there has been a rise in both the total sickbed numbers and number of medical professionals, but not in the number of people being diagnosed and treated. This means that the overall efficiency of the medical system is to be improved, and the same problem is also obvious as seen from the number of people diagnosed and treated by a doctor on average and the bed-utilization rate.

X. Chen
Department of Medical Ethics, Medical School of Shandong University, Shandong, China
e-mail: chenxy@sdu.edu.cn

J. Tao (ed.), *China: Bioethics, Trust, and the Challenge of the Market*,
© Springer Science+Business Media B.V. 2008

Table 1 The scale and efficiency of the health service system

Item \ Year	1990	2000	2002	2003
Total bed numbers of health establishments	2,925,390	3,177,000	3,136,110	3,164,022
Number of medical professionals	4,906,201	5,591,026	5,238,079	5,274,786
Number of the diagnosed or treated	25.59	21.23	21.45	20.96
Number of the diagnosed or treated by a doctor on average in provincial hospitals	unavailable	6.2	6.6	6.0
Number of the diagnosed or treated by a doctor on average in hospitals at the county level	unavailable	3.9	4.3	4.2
The bed utilization rate of general hospitals %	85.7	65	70.5	70.6
The bed utilization rate of hospitals in villages and towns %	43.4	33.2	34.9	36.3

2. Medical expenses have increased too quickly and people remain unsatisfied. In our interviews, the major belief among common people is that "it is too expensive to see a doctor". Table 2 illustrates the rise in medical costs in recent years.

A comparison between the results of two investigations on medical services, held in 1993 and 1998 gives a clear picture of the increase in the ratio of the sick people who do not go to a doctor after being ill for 2 weeks (see Table 3). About 38.2% of those who have been ill for 2 weeks do not go to a doctor because of economic difficulties (statistics of 2003).

Table 2 Average medical expenses (RMB Yuan)

Item \ Year	1995	2000	2002	2003
Average medical expenses of each outpatient in general hospitals (expressed in RMB Yuan)	39.9	85.8	99.6	108.2
Average medical expenses of each discharged in-patient in general hospitals (expressed in RMB Yuan)	1,667.8	3,083.7	3,597.7	3,910.7

Table 3 The rate of not going to a Doctor after being ill for 2 weeks (%)

	1993	1998	2003
The rate of not going to a doctor after being ill for 2 weeks %	36.4	38.5	48.9

In terms of satisfaction towards medical service, the data of the 2003 investigation on medical service demonstrates that the rate of non-dissatisfaction is 57.12%, and that 20.90% of the patients show great dissatisfaction towards medical costs (31.92% in urban and 17.58% in rural areas), which is the highest rate among all the most dissatisfactory items. Next to that, the most dissatisfactory items are the hospital facilities and environments, attitudes towards patients, complicated procedures, and the inconvenience of getting to hospitals.

An analysis of the supply and demand of medical resources reveals problems of both efficiency and quality, which has in turn impacted the utilization of medical resources, restrained people's demand, and made the whole medical system run at low efficiency. It is therefore quite necessary to further analyze the institution and mechanism of China's medical causes and probe into the approaches to improving the medical care situation.

2 The Character of Medical Service and Products, and the Function of the Market

Traditionally, people have always taken medical service as a kind of public good, directly produced and served by the government. However, in actuality, complete public goods in the real sense are very limited and a large number of products are exclusive. That is they have the characteristic of both public goods and private effects (Xu, 2003). It is especially so with medical services and medical products. Figure 1 shows the mixed character of medical services and products.

Furthermore, even public belongings have many possible supplying channels, such as pure governmental, private, and corporate partnerships. E. S. Savas has generalized ten specific modes of public service (Savas, 2000).

From an international perspective, there exists a clear trend toward privatizing public utilities. In many countries, governments have invited non-official and international capital to traditionally called public service, in order to attract financial resources other than those from the government to develop and provide, among other things, health service. The domestic market reform of NHS (National Health Services) in U.K. has separated the buyers from suppliers of the service and has introduced a competition mechanism into the traditional plan-controlled medical service. In the United States, with the rising of the tide of hospital reorganization in the 1990s, privately invested for-profit hospitals experienced the fastest development. In Germany, the leading characteristics in the reform of hospital systems has been greater play being given to private not-for-profit and for-profit hospitals.

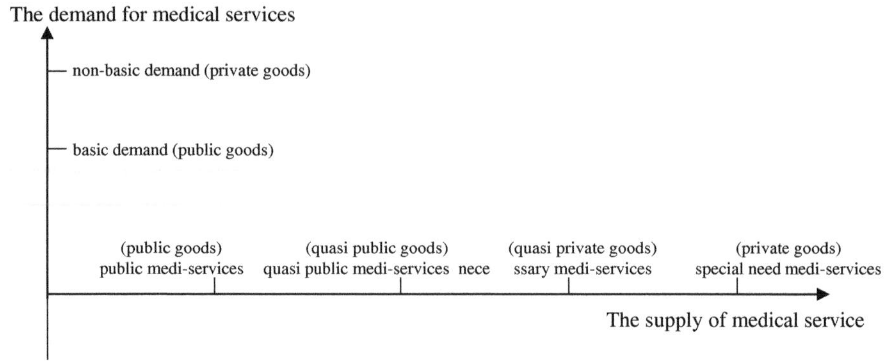

Fig. 1 The character of medical services and products

In Singapore, the major reform in public hospitals has been reorganization and the transfer of public hospitals, which used to be under the direct management of the Ministry of Health to self-supported health care companies. The function of the market can be summarized as follows:

1. The market serves to meet the various demands for health services. Private hospitals make up for the deficiency of public medical establishments by providing people with more choices in the following areas: specialized departments, geographic location, business hours, medical cost and diversified service to meet different needs.
2. The market constructs the micro-competition mechanism for health care services. The existence and development of private hospitals promote competition in the health care market, leads public hospitals to the quality of services and reduce the cost to the consumer.
3. The market guides the evolution of hospital operation and management. Generally speaking, public hospitals are slow to make changes; while private hospitals, free from many burdens, are more willing to be innovative. Research shows that the market mechanisms set up by private hospitals ensure that the administrative office serves the medical management and the medical management serves the patients, thus invigorating the health care market.
4. Developing private hospitals can motivate various active factors, make full use of all possible means, raise more health care funds, make up for the deficiency in medical resources and services in different places, better serve the people, and enhance the availability of health care services for people.

Through our interviews, we have determined that the advantages of private medical organizations are as follows: (1) comparatively low cost, (2) good service attitude, (3) convenient geographic location, (4) flexible and frequent hours, (5) simple treatment procedures, (6) diversified methods of payment, (7) better communication between doctors and patients, and (8) a better hospital environment.

In the 1990s, there was a striking rise in the health care provided by private capital in many countries (Yu & Zhang, 2002). China, after more than 20 years of reform, has established the framework of a market economic system. According to the plan of the state, by the year 2010, China will have established a fairly mature market economic system. Private establishments will likely be more important in the provision of China's health care service.

3 The Development of Private Hospitals in China

"Private hospital", a name we habitually use for a new type of hospital, originates from "private enterprises" and "private business", and represents a concept from the perspective of operational mechanisms. If a hospital is managed by the government, it is a public hospital or officially-run hospital. Otherwise, it is a private hospital. Public hospitals put stress on the role of a plan and government involvement in the distribution of medical resources and provision of health service, while private hospitals focus on the role of the market.

At the beginning of the founding of the People's Republic of China, apart from hospitals established by the government, there were a large numbers of individual doctors or independent private clinics. They became fewer and fewer until completely disappearing by the end of 1960s. Since the 1980s, with the implementation of various policies for reform and "opening up" and the progress in health care reform, private clinics were allowed to open business again. In the 1990s, privately invested hospitals and joint or cooperative hospitals with foreign partners also emerged, and the situation of hospitals run by diversified investment started to take shape. In 2001, with the implementation of the policy to manage hospitals according to their different types, private hospitals got their appropriate and justified position. Henceforth, private hospitals have experienced prompt development, and a large amount of social capital in an investment zone that was previously restricted.

According to statistics, right now there are 1,500 private hospitals of different types in China. The rise of this force has broken the complete monopoly of the health care market by public hospitals, and has refilled the health care market with energy and fresh air. However, if compared with the more than 70,000 state-owned hospitals, which constitute the main stream of the medical system, private hospitals are far from being substantially influential. In 2001, the Statistics and Information Center of the Ministry of Public Health announced that the private hospitals in Guangdong took 39.12% of the total medical establishments, and the figures in Shanghai, Zhejiang and Fujian were 15.9%, 53.22% and 59.98%, respectively (Huang & Liang, 2003). It can be seen that in terms of quantity, private hospitals have taken a comparatively large proportion. However, another group data shows a huge gap between private hospitals and state-owned ones in terms of business scale and medical service actually provided by them. Certified doctors in private hospitals only made up 2.74% of the national total; certified nurses, 2.19%; outpatients,

3.06%; discharged inpatients, 2.84%; and emergency treatment to critical cases, 2.19%. The use rate of beds in private hospitals was 50.6%, lower than the 64.6% of state-owned hospitals (Liu et al., 2004).

A study made by the School of Public Health of Beijing University indicates that the general satisfaction rate by outpatients over their last visits to private hospitals is 72.7%, and to private clinics is 76.7%, higher than that to public hospitals and public clinics, which registers 54.4% and 64.9%, respectively. The usual reason for dissatisfaction at public hospitals and clinics is "ineffective treatment", which accounts for 46% of the dissatisfaction rate, followed by "expensive medical cost", which accounts for 31%. The residents' appraisals of private medical organizations were higher than those of public medical organizations when asked about the following characteristics: the position of clinics, waiting time, doctors' explanation of the diseases and diagnosis, the respect for and care of patients, the rational degree of the cost, etc. However, when asked about the hospital environment, medical treatment skills and the selection of doctors, public medical organizations won better appraisals than private medical organizations (Zhang et al., 2003). A research result by the Department of Public Health of Zhejiang Province also shows that almost every patient was satisfied with the service attitude of the medical professionals in private hospitals and clinics and these hospitals and clinics charge at an average or even at lower prices as compared with public ones.

Undoubtedly, there remain quite a few problems in the development of private hospitals such as: (1) the overall quality of medical treatment pending for improvement, (2) the unclear orientation of hospital development, (3) low efficiency in using the resources, (4) irrational treatment and use of medicine and over-treatment in some private hospitals, (5) unfair competition, and (6) the overstatement of the curative effect to mislead patients. In management, they suffer from incomplete systemization, insufficient administrative proficiency, and lacking exploration and innovation in management concept, business operation and management measures. In addition, the low quality of the medical professionals also restrains a robust development of private hospitals as well (Yang, 2002).

4 An Analysis on the External and Internal Scenario of Private Hospitals in China

Presently, the number of private medical establishments in China has grown considerably. During the health care reform, the classification and corresponding management of for-profit and not-for-profit hospitals also predict a further advancement of private medical establishments. However, our research results so far point out many imminent issues facing the development of private hospitals in China.

1. Private hospitals have difficulty in being appointed as designated hospitals for treatment in the medical care insurance scheme.

In the view of the law and regulations such as Interim Provisions on Designated Medical Establishments for Treatment in the Basic Medical Care Insurance Scheme, there is no exclusion of for-profit hospitals. The essential criteria for getting the approval lie in the service charge and service quality. Any legal medical establishment can become a designated hospital, so long as it meets the requirement to give treatment to beneficiaries who reimburse their medical cost from the basic medical care insurance scheme in service quality and charge standard, and passes the examination carried out by administrative organizations for medical and health care. The directors of some for-profit hospitals have stated privately that it is difficult for private hospitals to get the approval necessary to be included in the health care insurance system.

2. Private hospitals are facing greater business costs and operational risks.
   The not-for-profit medical establishments owned by the government enjoy favorable tax policies in addition to getting financial support from relevant government organizations, while private hospitals can only survive in a very narrow space of the medical market, because, apart from running into great operational risks, they must confront obscure policies on taxation, insurance and so forth. The president of a private hospital in Jinan said during the interview, "In terms of business scope and strength, we are by no means able to compete with large scale state-owned hospitals, which are facilitated by advanced equipment, comprehensive specialized departments and strong financial support. Furthermore, taking the overall business environment into account, we are facing greater costs and risks."
3. Private hospitals as a whole lack market competitiveness
   Most of the private hospitals today are: (a) small in scale, (b) simple in structure, (c) have a small market share, (d) limited in medical service and (e) lack the technology and personnel found in public hospitals. In most cases, the specialized departments set up by many private hospitals are for short-term purposes, thereby causing these hospitals to have a less competitive edge than big public hospitals with high-tech content service items. Moreover, for most private hospitals, service items and business scope are limited by insufficient financial input, and by obsolete equipment, simple and crude facilities, and uneven medical proficiency.
4. Private hospitals are short of talented personnel
   Our research shows that 90% of persons looking for work in the health care industry would choose state-owned and not-for-profit hospitals. State-owned and non-profit hospitals are recognized and are known for carrying out research and for providing medical education. Consequently, such hospitals may attract many outstanding people who prefer research and available teaching positions rather than economic benefits. Therefore, private hospitals find themselves in an inferior position to public hospitals. During an interview, the president of a private hospital in Jinan said, "We hope the state can back up the development of private hospitals by providing personnel and financial support and by giving a better and more comfortable space for development."

5 Solutions and Suggestions for the Development of Private Hospitals in China

To meet the medical demand of various circles, competition in medical services is the key. However, without supporting policies and an environment for fair competition, nobody will make the investment, pioneer the service sectors, or improve service quality. To this end, it is imperative to develop policies and an environment to encourage competition during the course of health care reform. With regard to the problems existing in the development of private hospitals in China, this thesis makes the following solutions and suggestions:

First, efforts should be made in reforming the health care system and spurring diversification and fair competition. It is important to create a situation where medical establishments of various ownerships and levels can co-exist. At the present stage, the Chinese government should, on the one hand, re-vision the function and orientation of public hospitals, focus financial support to a limited number of key hospitals and rationally allocate some "affordable hospitals" in order to assure basic medical and health care and safeguard the fairness of health care service. On the other hand, the government should give incentives to other investors to build for-profit and not-for-profit medical establishments and "let go" and privatize those public hospitals, which are beyond the obligations and capacity of the government. As a result, incentives will be given to fair and diversified competition to enhance quality and constrain cost. The fact is, only by investing over 30 million can one establish a general hospital with basically complete facilities. The best practice now is to make an investment into a present hospital or make an acquisition, namely, "borrowing a shell" instead of establishing a new hospital (Yang, 2002).

Second, encouragement should be given to the development of high standard, private hospitals. Many researches and investigations indicate that the weakest point of private establishments is their substandard professional competency. This also explains why patients still resort to public hospitals for cardiovascular diseases. In line with the actual situation of classified hospital registration in China, we reckon that full play should be given to institutional innovation to contain medical cost and to improve the quality of services, and that the development of more private hospitals should be encouraged to further invigorate competition. For instance, incentives should be given to non-official capital to make various investments in building new private hospitals. In the meantime, efforts should be made to close, stop, or merge some public hospitals and convert some of them into private hospitals. The medical professionals of private hospitals should be increased and improved as a supplement to the needs of the Chinese medical system and as a vital force of the new medical system. In terms of policy support, private hospitals should share the same treatment with state-owned hospitals, and institutional barriers that hinder the sound development of private economy should be lifted. Equal treatment should be given to private hospitals in the designation as hospitals for medical insurance, in the promotion of the doctors' professional ranks and titles, in academic activities and in personnel cultivation.

Thirdly, the taxation policy to private hospitals should be appropriately adjusted and improved. At present, an overwhelming number of regions classify for-profit hospitals as a service sector and levy 5% of the business volume as business tax. According to the provisions in tax-related laws, business tax shall be calculated as part of the cost, and the cost of the hospital will be increased due to the hand-over of business tax. The increased cost can be digested in two ways: one is to increase service charges in order to pass the costs onto patients, and the other is for the private hospitals themselves to take measures to solve the cost problem by reducing service costs by lowering service quality or by giving up the basic but low profit service items. Obviously we do not prefer to take either of these measures. However, only by eliminating the business tax for medical services can there be a fair competition scenario. In addition, while fulfilling its duty-free commitments in 3 years, the government should offer medical organizations a favorable tax policy, which is different from those that pertain to industry and commerce. A tax deduction should be given to cover those expenditures, which aim to (a) improve patients' medical treatment conditions, (b) prevent epidemics, and (c) reduce the medical expenses of impoverished patients.

Fourth, efforts should be made to strengthen supervision and control over private hospitals to enhance their overall prestige. At the initial stage, private hospitals in China have made some progress, but also have encountered many problems. Many of the people that we interviewed mentioned the problem of qualification and proficiency of the medical professionals in private hospitals. In some private hospitals, doctors with genuine or false qualifications or proficiencies are mixed together and many people without formal medical education are conducting medical practice. The pursuit of short-term, economic profit has caused many misdiagnoses or therapeutic errors. In some private hospitals, the problem of selling fake medicine is very serious. Other problems include false advertisements, fraudulent publicity of doctors' professional ranks and titles, exaggerated curative effect, over-treatment, and equipment shortage. Many medical professionals working in private hospitals complain that illegal medical practices have created a misunderstanding among people about legal and standard medical establishments. Therefore, we strongly suggest that the government strengthen its supervision and management over private medical establishments in order to protect the patients' medical safety in earnest, and to further enhance the overall prestige of private medical establishments.

References

Huang, C., & Liang, H. (2003). A study on the non-governmental health organizations. In *China Health Care Management*, No. 7.

Liu, D., Fengwen, Liu, T., & Chi, B. (2004). Research report on policy environment of for-profit hospitals. In *Chinese Hospitals*, No. 5.

Savas, E. S. (2000). *Privatization and public–private partnerships* (pp. 70–88). New York: Chatham House. (Chinese translation: China People's University Press).

Xu, B. (2003, December). *Introduction to public economics* (p.112). Ha erbin: Heilongjiang People's Publishing House, No. 5.

Yang, Q. (2002). Upon the orientation of private hospital development. In *Hygienic Economics Study*, No. 3.

Yu, M., & Zhang, X. (2002). A study on the private health care in developing countries. In *Foreign Medicine: Hospital Management*, No. 3.

Zhang, T., Yanghui, Fengwen, Zhou, Z., Chen, Y., & Lin, M. (2003, September). An outline of the function and scope of private health care in China. In *China Hospital Management Journal*, No. 3, 527–530.

China, Beware: What American Health Care Has to Learn from Singapore

H. Tristram Engelhardt, Jr.*

1 Introduction: What the Market Is and What It Is Not

The market is freedom. The market is nothing more than men and women consentingly trading goods and services. The market in general, since it binds persons across the world who are often to each other moral strangers, can require only that those involved give permission. That is, they can be required not to coerce by threat of force or through deception. Such challenges to the market fall beyond the capacity of the market itself and must be met through rule of law. The problem of physical necessity also falls beyond the scope of the market. Concerns to blunt such necessity must be met by altruism. Finally, the market takes for granted that, though its participants may enter into the marketplace for numerous reasons, the most common reason is the desire for profit. The moral domestication of concerns for profit will need to take place through moral institutions and through frameworks of moral concern that lie beyond the market. One should expect from the market only that which the market can provide.

Human history, especially the history of the twentieth century, has shown the powerful, innovative force of the market. The market inspires discovery. In complex ways, it brings men and women together and motivates them to invent new products and services. This is also a cardinal feature of the health care markets. Innovation in pharmaceuticals and medical devices has come from the desire for profit. It promises the amelioration of a wide range of morbidity and mortality risks. The market also produces wealth. It increases the amount of resources available, which in and of themselves decrease morbidity and mortality risks, for poverty is associated with early death and more suffering. Finally, the market is an efficient distributor of goods and services. The twentieth century has shown the global failure of centrally-planned markets to meet the needs and desires of their citizens. No

H.T. Engelhardt Jr., M.D., Ph.D.
Professor of Philosophy, Rice University, and Professor Emeritus, Baylor College of Medicine
e-mail: htengelh@rice.edu

* He is Editor of the *Journal of Medicine and Philosophy*, the Philosophy and Medicine book series, and Senior Editor of the journal *Christian Bioethics*, as well as the book series Philosophical Studies in Contemporary Culture.

J. Tao (ed.), *China: Bioethics, Trust, and the Challenge of the Market*,

© Springer Science+Business Media B.V. 2008

central, rational point of view can approach the rapidity and nuanced character of the market in its responses to shifting desires and resource availability. In short, the market is a powerful source of goods and services. It spurs innovation, creates wealth, and efficiently distributes goods and services.

The market is not everything. The market is not a way in which one usually responds out of love or consideration to others. If one attends only to the concerns of the market, one's life will be radically one-sided and incomplete, if not morally perverse. The whole human being has, or at least should have, a wide range of interests and concerns beyond those of becoming richer and having more resources. Besides pursuing profit, one should act out of generosity and love. It should therefore come as no surprise that the market does not exhaust the range of human concerns, or that it must be supplemented by altruistic interests in other human beings, including the pursuit of the good of one's own family, friends, and strangers. The turn to altruism is itself not enough. Humans must also establish the effective rule of law: humans are often weak of will and moved by inordinate passions of greed, lust, and aggression. As a consequence, human activities must be constrained so that some humans do not use other humans without their permission. The rule of law is also essential to enforce contracts and to punish deception: fraud and breach of contract undermine the freedom of agreements. The trinity of market, altruism, and law must be rightly balanced, so that each can realize fully that which is within its scope. Only if the market, altruism, and the law do that which they can do well can persons fully pursue human flourishing.

In society in general and health care in particular, one must know whom and what institutions one can trust and for what. For example, one can trust the market to produce new pharmaceuticals and devices that will reduce morbidity and mortality risks, and to increase wealth, which itself will reduce morbidity and mortality risks. One can trust the market in general to be a much more efficient means for distributing most goods and services than governments. However, one cannot trust the market to motivate altruism. The roots of altruism need to be found elsewhere. Since all altruism is concrete, the nurturing of altruism will require concrete communities with concrete understandings of the good and therefore of beneficence and human flourishing.[1] To stress a previous point once again: protection against violence, coercion, and deception cannot be sought in the market, but must be sought in the rule of law. It is a foundational and misleading confusion to expect from the market what altruism and the rule of law must. If one faults the market for not producing that which is beyond its scope, one has made a category mistake.

China needs institutions it can trust. As China moves to the future, it will need to trust in a market that is free enough to produce the innovative breakthroughs through which China will benefit its own people, as well as become rich through benefiting others. It will need to trust in a market that is free enough from external interventions so as to raise the standard of living for all Chinese and to distribute goods and services efficiently. While recognizing all the benefits the market has to offer, China must appreciate the ways in which failure to support the rule of law and altruism-supporting institutions such as the family will distort the market through no fault of the market. In particular, Chinese policymakers will need to recognize the importance of nurturing those institutions that support altruism and charity.

A proper emphasis on the rule of law should not be confused with intrusive regulations that distort the functioning of the market and, despite the best of intentions, corrupt medical practice. As noted by Benfu Li (Li, 2006), there is a widespread practice of providing physicians with cash payments (i.e., red packets) so as to acquire better quality care or access to a better qualified physician. This practice occurs because the fees for physician services are held artificially low, inducing all physicians to seek extra payments. In addition, there is not an easy market mechanism to pay more for better health services. The appearance of the black-market practice of red packets is thus not an expression of a market failure, but of the distorting influence of well-meaning but corrupting regulations. The same is the case with another response to the low fees set for physicians. Unlike North America and most European countries, in China physicians not only prescribe medications, but they sell them as well. When physician fees are frozen at an artificially low level but there is an opportunity to supplement one's income with profits from the sale of medications, there will be a temptation to prescribe more medication than needed or more expensive pharmaceuticals than needed. These corrupting pressures on the clinical judgment are not a result of a market failure, nor are they the direct result of the corrupt attitude of physicians, but instead are the result of distorting regulations. One will have made a crucial mistake if one blames the market for failures in altruism or for the distortion to the market due to the overreaching of government rules and regulations.

As the market begins to play an ever larger role in Chinese health care, it will be important for China to avoid the mistakes and problems besetting health care policy in North America and Western Europe. Central to an appreciation of the difficulties will be recognizing clearly when they have been breaches of trust. Rather than trusting in intermediary institutions that can sustain thick understandings of altruism, North American and Western European polities to various extents have focused on establishing thick webs of governmentally supported entitlements to health care often set within a robustly egalitarian ethos. The first has led to unsustainable commitments on the part of governments to provide health care, much of which has been the product of the political hazard of promising entitlements in the present that will need to be funded in the future, thus disconnecting promises from the responsibility to keep the promises. Here, trust in government has proven false. In addition, egalitarian commitments have led to radical restrictions of individual market freedoms in Canada and to the failure to embrace health care or medical savings accounts, which can help avoid political and moral hazards.

2 Moral and Political Hazards

The United States and other Western democracies have failed to develop a sustainable approach to financing health care: health care expenditures have risen absolutely and as a percentage of the gross domestic product,[2] while unfunded entitlements to health care have been created for a growing elderly population.[3] The result is a major and growing breech of societal and public trust. In part, this is a result of a failure to reward responsible personal choices in the purchase of health care services. In part, it is also a result of the role played by government in mandating particular benefit packages,[4] as well as through policies that make the provision of health care a non-taxed benefit for employees (National Center for Policy Analysis, 1995). Core to the difficulties have been commitments to the creation of health care entitlements and an egalitarian ideology. This paper indicates a way out of these difficulties by offering a suggestion that reflects elements of Singapore's approach to health care financing.[5]

Although reference is made to Singapore and although there are many similarities between this proposal and practices in Singapore, the suggestions here depart in many ways from actual Singaporean policy. The policy outlined here takes seriously family-oriented, responsible, private choice through the development of health care savings plans that allow cost- and asset-shifting within families. It focuses on the goal of avoiding the dangers of an egalitarian ideology and the creation of unfunded entitlements, which undermine the long-term sustainability of any health care system. It recognizes as well that these untoward outcomes require the symbolic and moral resources of a civil society with substantive cultural resources sustained within an association formed an institution intermediate between individuals and the states.

All health care systems are beset by the problem that the desire for services exceeds available budgets, leading to an upward spiral of health care costs. American and Western European attempts to frame a coherent moral basis for a health care policy that provides all citizens with basic coverage, encourages innovation, and contains costs have failed. For example, there has been a failure to come to terms with the circumstance that any attempt to cap profits in the development of pharmaceuticals and medical devices tends to slow innovation and therefore advantage patients in the present over against patients in the future. The profits made by the pharmaceutical and medical-device industries tend to be regarded with envy and without the appreciation that (1) absent such profits to drive innovation, not only will the development of new ways of reducing morbidity and mortality risks be postponed, but as in the case of new threats such as SARS and avian flu, one may fail to find ways of countering such dangers in time to avoid significant global tragedies. (2) Absent marked profits for the pharmaceutical and medical-device industries, capital investment will shift to other industries where significant profits will not be regarded as improper (e.g., the production of video games). The unpleasant fact of the matter is that some must get better treatment first so that all can have better treatment sooner in the future. A dynamic and innovative health care system will be inegalitarian.

This paper therefore begins with the background recognition that, while medical advances offer the prospect of lowering morbidity and mortality risks through the development of ever more effective health care interventions, they at the same time generate more costs, at least in the short run. Second, egalitarian health care systems such as Canada's can never provide all citizens with all health care services from which they might benefit and therefore must limit the private purchase of health care (Graham, 2008). Such approaches remove incentives for health care users to learn how prudently to make choices as to which health care interventions at what costs are worth what benefits for them. Such systems tend not to reward new and often initially costly health care innovations. Last, if there is good evidence to indicate that market forces are crucial not only for the efficient distribution of goods and services, including medical goods and services, but also for spurring medical innovation in a medical market that has now become international, then the market and private health care will need to be taken seriously.

When considering how these reflections bear on China and the bioethical challenges it faces, one must note that, just like the developed countries of Europe and North America, China will confront three cardinal challenges to the stability of its health care system. First, developed countries are characterized by an increasing proportion of their population living beyond retirement age and therefore no longer contributing payments for their health care expenses. Second, an ever larger portion of this population is significantly advanced in age (e.g., over 80) so as to be in particular need of high-intensity health care interventions. Third, there is a decreasing portion of the population in the workforce providing the funds to support health care not only for themselves but also for the retired, the physiologically brittle, and the vulnerable aged. China has the advantage of being able to consider in advance about how it will respond to limited resources and rising costs in the face of the promises of innovation so as to avoid the health care policy problems currently besetting North America and Europe.

In countries still under development, this cluster of challenges is further complicated by three other issues. First, there are internal geographical disparities in health care resources so that attempts to achieve anything close to equal availability of resources across the country cannot be realized by leveling up, since the resources available are limited. An attempt to level up would be financially unsustainable. Second, the attempt to achieve an equal availability of services can therefore only be achieved through dramatic governmental constraints aimed at leveling down the quality and also likely the quantity of services available in regions marked by higher levels of development. One would need to define the concept of basic health care downward and forbid those with resources to buy better basic care. As a consequence, attempts to achieve equality across the country would be made at the price of lowering the support for innovation in parts of China where there is a concentration of expertise and resources. Third, attempts to create equal availability of health care through leveling down of services would also provide significant incentives for physicians with talent to go elsewhere to pursue their professional goals, and patients with resources to go elsewhere to seek their health care. Such policies would not only disable centers of excellence and innovation, but export the talent needed for China's future. Though attempts to level down even in developed countries have the untoward effects noted above (e.g., Canada), matters are made more difficult in countries that are becoming old before they are rich, in comparison to countries that became rich before a large proportion of their population became old.

This complex cluster of challenges to health care policy defines the context for China as it moves (1) to provide an adequate level of care for all its citizens, (2) to achieve an appropriate balance between the roles of the government, private investment, and the market, and (3) to develop a successful and innovative health care system and biomedical industry. As China begins to reclaim its global economic leadership, it will need to examine critically the bioethical foundations it should embrace for its health care system and turn to those traditional cultural resources that will support responsible behavior and choice.

3 The Foundations of Bioethics Critically Reconsidered

As a field of scholarship and practice under the name bioethics, biomedical moral reflection is now entering its fourth decade.[6] Though scholarship has matured and important intellectual programs are in place, two circumstances have not been honestly faced. First, there is no common agreement regarding a particular moral vision that should guide bioethics. There is no global bioethics. Second and more importantly, one can understand why this is the case, in that any particular moral account requires establishing as canonical a particular ranking of cardinal goods and right-making conditions. That is, establishing any particular moral view as canonical requires granting a background foundation such that the establishment of any particular concrete account inevitably begs the question, argues in a circle, or engages in infinite regress.[7] The recognition of this difficulty, for example, is reflected in the retreat of John Rawls from the project of advancing a particular, morally normative view that can then in turn justify a particular system of allocating health care resources.[8] In the face of irreconcilable moral diversity, bioethics has instead had success in developing procedural approaches that rely on authorization from the participants, rather than reference to a canonical moral vision.[9]

By default, since bioethics is left with a health care policy that relies for its authority on the authorization of its participants, the cardinal practices turn out to be the use of contracts, the market, and limited constitutional democracies. These allow for the emergence and flourishing of private associations and institutions such as characterize both for-profit and not-for-profit hospitals and health care systems. Not only does one find private health care and market forces to be salient and successful, but one can as well understand the moral justification for this state of affairs. In addition, one can appreciate the moral importance of particular institutions framing their own moral character and integrity. They are the natural outcome of persons through common agreement entering into the provision of health care. By joining together around and through particular thick views of virtuous medical practice, they nest the market delivery of health care within a set of strong moral commitments. If individuals are allowed in free association to fashion health care institutions and systems that reflect their own particular moral commitments, then thick understandings of morality can take on a communal life that can support substantive appreciations of honesty, trustworthiness, and charity.

In the West, such thick moral communal understandings have been found most frequently associated with religiously affiliated hospitals. However, one can as well imagine hospitals established around Confucian cultural-moral commitments.[10]

Since all accounts of the good are particular, in order to pursue virtue one must be embedded within particular moral communities with their concrete moral perspectives. China will need to explore the cultural resources it possesses that can support trust and reliability in the delivery of health care. It is the presence of such communities with their treasury of moral and symbolic resources that can make responsible choice possible.

4 Facing Finitude

The United States, Canada, Europe, and indeed all countries, including China, are faced with the challenge of financing health care for their citizens. The difficulties lie not simply in the ways in which providers are available to offer health care, or in the ways in which services are financed, but also in the very character of human finitude. All health care systems confront the following unpleasant circumstances:

1. all humans will die;
2. all humans who do not die at once will suffer before they die;
3. most humans wish to ameliorate their suffering and postpone their death;
4. as the proportion of a country's population over retirement age (and especially those over 80 likely needing long-term care and high-cost medical interventions) increases, the use of health care and its costs increase;
5. however, health care can only marginally reduce but not eliminate suffering and only marginally postpone death;
6. the marginal reduction of suffering and postponement of death is ever more costly at the margins;
7. resources for the support of health care are limited;
8. humans disagree as to what should count as an appropriate, just, fair, or even basic allocation of health care resources, in that human, secular, moral, epistemological resources are insufficient to establish a particular, canonical, content-full, moral vision through sound rational argument;
9. because medical knowledge tends to be probabilistic, and because humans have different understandings of what should count as appropriate allocations of health care resources, persons as well as health care systems must decide in the face of uncertainty and moral controversy what investments of resources at what likelihood of success are worthwhile;
10. because there are only three ways to attract resources (namely, love, coercion, and the search for profit) and because there are limits to altruism and to the willingness to be taxed, the appeal to profit will play a cardinal role in all effective health care systems;
11. insofar as increased taxation is associated with decreased societal productivity, and insofar as the profit motive is necessary to spur innovation in general and medical innovation in particular (e.g., the production of new pharmaceuticals and medical devices), societies will learn by bitter experience the costs of overtaxing and limiting profits in the medical-industrial complex;

12. as a result, different societies will establish different approaches to defining what basic health care should be provided to those in need and under what circumstances: health care policy and the bioethics that underlies it are irremediably diverse.

This state of affairs guarantees that health care will always tend to be distributed unequally, that attempts to restrain the market will impose costs related to fewer innovations and a lower quality of basic care, and that there will be diverse strategies to come to terms with this circumstance. This state of affairs is embedded in the character of medical resource scarcity, which guarantees that there will always be a demand for ever more health care, and that since resources are limited this will tend to divert ever more resources from other undertakings to health care. A health care financing system that is successful must in one way or the other induce individuals to forego high-cost, low-yield treatment and to invest resources towards other goals.

All health care financing systems confront powerful forces that tend to drive up expenditures for health care. These include:

1. Moral hazards generated by patients being given entitlements to services: once an entitlement is in the hands of a patient, the patient or the patient's family will tend to use it to the utmost, even when such use may not be either prudent or cost-effective, because this imposes on them no further costs.
2. Political hazards engendered by the temptation of politicians to create non-fully-funded entitlements for patients, with the result that legislation is enacted that promises benefits that will need to be funded by future tax payments, economic growth, etc. (these political hazards in particular mark media democracies, where politicians are tempted to gain election or advance their political careers through promising overly generous health care entitlements as well as unfeasible egalitarian systems)
3. Scientific and technological advances, though desired by most for better protection against or relief from morbidity and mortality risks, are often initially expensive and available only to a few.

Any health care system that would both contain costs and support innovation will need to come to terms with these significant moral and public policy challenges.

The United States have failed to contain health care costs successfully, because they have failed to embrace an ideology that can contain the moral and political hazards that beset health care financing. Instead, the United States have generally tacitly embraced an ideology[11] that promises

1. the best of care to all,
2. equal care to all, and
3. cost containment.

Of course, these three goals are mutually at tension. In particular, this ideology is incompatible with cost containment, the support of innovation, and the development of the virtue of responsible decision-making. This ideology has also made it difficult for Americans to pursue a coherent use of private resources and private health care institutions. This ideology has made it difficult as well for America coherently to engage the strengths of private health care institutions and private health care choices.

In contrast, in order to confront the challenges of health care financing, a system must be embraced that

1. promises to all some basic health care, but not the best basic care,
2. acknowledges that health care will be unequally available, while
3. making patients and their families recognize the cost of these health care services
4. through encouraging responsible, individual choice.

To contain health care costs, one must learn to live with inequalities, because persons and families will have different health care needs, different financial resources, and different levels of willingness to forgo some health care so as to retain resources for other purposes. One will need to explore how to aid patients in embracing an ethos of responsible choice. One will need to favor practices that reward value-oriented resource accumulation.

For this to be successful, the market and medicine must be embedded in framing institutions that provide thick, symbolic, moral points of reference, as well as grounds to motivate reliable and trustworthy action. At the very least, there must be structures that

1. sustain commitments to the rule of law,
2. nurture a sense of professionalism on the part of physicians,
3. strengthen commitments to those structures in society such as families, and communities formed around particular understandings of human flourishing that nurture concrete visions of free and responsible choice and motivate altruism.

The presence of such institutions and social structures is necessary to direct the market towards appropriate goals and away from unacceptable harms to patients, the medical profession, and families. For example, to ensure that pharmaceutical and medical advertisements are honest and not misleading, the rule of law must secure appropriate punishment for fraudulent statements. More important yet, there must be structures within the society that can draw on its traditional moral commitments, so as to present effective visions of virtuous conduct in the market, as well as altruism in the practice of medicine.

5 The Building Blocks of Health Care Financing Systems

At the outset, one must distinguish among health care systems that have one or more of the following sorts of providers.

1. private, for-profit providers, including both individual practitioners, hospitals, and corporations formed to provide health care;
2. private, not-for-profit providers, including individual practitioners, hospitals, and corporations formed to provide health care;

3. governmental entities, including both hospitals and health care systems that, though governmental, are local and may still compete among each other as well as with private for-profit and not-for-profit providers in attracting patients and physicians;
4. unified governmental systems that provide health care.

Within one country, all of the above entities can exist and in various ways compete with each other for patients. An example of such a complex arrangement is offered by the United States, where there are private for-profit, private not-for-profit, and various local government-supported hospital systems that can compete with each other, as well as country-wide systems such as the Veterans health care system (e.g., providing services under certain circumstances for individuals who served in the US armed forces). The first three allow the benefits of market competition, while the first two can in different ways attract capital and support innovation (though technically non-profit institutions do not produce profits, they can and often do produce excess funds, which can richly reward the institution's management).

There are as well a number of ways to structure the payment of providers, whether private for-profit, not-for-profit, or governmental. These involve greater or lesser private control of the resources used in the purchase of health care. At the outset, one must distinguish among possible payment systems, including those in which

1. patients themselves are expected on their own both to save for their health care expenditures and to pay for them; this is the approach to many out-of-hospital care in Hong Kong;
2. patients are constrained to save for themselves and then to pay for their own health care either from their usual disposable resources or from specially established savings accounts, though they may deploy the funds in such savings accounts for purposes other than health care, should resources remain after such purchases; such savings accounts can be distinguished by special family-friendly characteristics that allow the sharing of these resources without tax consequences;
3. patients who are impecunious are provided by the government with funds in a special savings account into which the patients are also required to contribute, insofar as they have earnings, and from which they can purchase health care, although they may deploy the funds for purposes other than health care, should resources remain after such purchases; such savings accounts can be distinguished by special family-friendly characteristics that allow the sharing of these resources without tax consequences;
4. patients are at liberty to purchase various insurance packages that will retrospectively pay for the health care that patients in the future choose to purchase;
5. patients are at liberty to purchase various insurance packages that seek to contain costs through managing in various prospective fashions the ways in which health expenditures are incurred through determining in advance which health

care providers may be used and/or which services can in particular circumstances be purchased;
6. the employers of patients purchase various insurance packages that will retrospectively pay for the health care patients choose to purchase in the future;
7. the employers of patients purchase various insurance packages but seek to contain costs through managing in various prospective fashions the ways in which health expenditures are incurred by determining in advance which health care providers may be used and/or which services can in particular circumstances be purchased under the insurance plan;
8. government entities create tax-supported entitlements, either directly or through vouchers, to retrospective reimbursement for the health care patients choose to purchase;
9. government entities create tax-supported entitlements to health care, either directly or through vouchers, but attempt to contain costs by determining in advance which health care providers may be used and/or which services can be purchased in particular circumstances.

Health care financing schemes that provide entitlements to health care, even when costs are controlled through prospective management systems, find themselves under pressure of increases in expenditure. Once entitlements are in place, users usually attempt to extract maximally all the services they can, thus leading to various co-payment schemes.

Only the first three approaches to health care financing (direct private purchase, private purchase from mandatory savings accounts, and private purchase from governmental-augmented mandatory savings accounts) can provide incentives for patients to avoid the moral hazard of over-using entitlements, as well as for politicians to avoid the political hazard of legislating unfunded entitlements. The second and the third can support family cohesion, collaboration, and altruism if the resources can be transferred without tax consequences to family members for health care as well as retirement needs. That is, one can support the social stability of a society by inducing family members to save and collaborate. Such savings schemes can be further buttressed by catastrophic health care insurance. In order to establish a sustainable health care system, one must abandon an egalitarian ideology and take seriously nurturing an ethos of responsible choice by putting into place practices that reward resource accumulation for health care, as well as other purposes.[12]

6 Some Tentative Conclusions: Shaping a Bioethics that Takes Responsibility and Property Rights Seriously

These reflections on the challenges of fashioning a sustainable health care financing scheme support the conclusion that a financially feasible policy must counter the role of value orientations that undercut the possibility of long-term financial stability. In this regard, three points critical of current policies deserve special emphasis:

1. an entitlement mentality should be avoided –
   a. the affirmation of health care entitlements is fraught with moral hazards, in that once entitlements are created, they tend to be used to their utmost by patients and the families of patients, thus consuming inordinate amounts of resources;
   b. the affirmation of health care entitlements is also fraught with political hazards, in that the ability to create unfunded entitlements can be used by politicians in media democracies to secure re-election and advance their careers, thus creating burdens for future generations;
2. the affirmation of an egalitarian ideology should be avoided –
   a. egalitarian ideologies dampen innovation in limiting health care investments so that, as a result, capital is not available for the development of new and innovative technologies;
   b. egalitarian ideologies undercut individual and family responsibility in making health care choices;
3. the establishment of an entitlement mentality or an egalitarian ideology should be avoided –
   a. the coercive imposition of an entitlement mentality collides with private property rights, as well as responsible resource accumulation and use in being focused primarily on transfer payments in order to support the entitlements created;[13]
   b. the coercive imposition of an egalitarian ideology collides with the basic right to dispose of one's private property in the peaceable pursuit with consenting others of a vision of human flourishing.

Given the inability of bioethics to justify through sound rational argument a particular moral vision as canonical, these conclusions not only accord with that which is financially sustainable, but reflect as well the moral state of affairs in which we find ourselves as we fashion health care policy. It is not possible to provide through sound rational argument the general moral authority needed to establish encompassing egalitarian- or entitlement-oriented policies. The justification of such totalizing regimes is beyond secular moral justification. By default, we are left with individuals and their choices as primary.

It was out of a recognition of the limits of secular moral rationality that both the United States and Texas framed limited democratic understandings of political governance through formal-right constitutions. In particular, they eschewed assertions of entitlement-directed claims integral to material-right constitutions. It is the latter combined with an egalitarian ideology that have undergirded social-democratic understandings expressed in the Canadian commitment to equality in health care through leveling all down to a constrained standard of basic health care choices. Such approaches to theory and health care policy are at the heart of political theories such as those of John Rawls (Rawls, 1971) and of concerns for health care policy, as endorsed by Norman Daniels (Daniels, 1985). These theories, when realized within constitutional frameworks and policies for the delivery of health care, presuppose a thin theory of the good, which assumes a particular ranking of human moral concerns, such that civil libertarian interests trump those of equality of opportunity and those of equality of opportunity trump those of prosperity. As the latter Rawls conceded, this thin theory of the good and it's ranking of values is not grounded in a general rational necessity, but in a particular understanding of an appropriate constitutional framework (Rawls, 1993).

The inability to establish the moral authority for egalitarian- or entitlement-oriented policies by default justifies a limited democratic approach to constitutionalism and health care policy. However, in circumstances where overall political stability is a significant concern, it may be possible to justify a fiduciary market polity that gives accent first to security rights and then to market rights, and only then to the civil libertarian claims of a limited formal-right constitution. If such is the case, one can then place directed fiduciary market polities[14] between social-democratic constitutional states and limited democratic states in terms of their general moral plausibility. In particular, one can see why approaches to governance and to health care financing, as one finds in Singapore, are morally much more easily defended than approaches such as Canada. The latter, though it in general allows greater civil libertarian rights, nevertheless more starkly limits property rights. With Hegel, one can appreciate the priority of property rights as core to the incarnate human person (Hegel, *The Philosophy of Right*, §54), who is the source of secular moral authority.

The recognition of this state of affairs can serve as a basis for establishing a financially sustainable approach to health care through strengthening property rights in resources for health care through establishing individual health care savings accounts. In order to prevent the danger associated with establishing egalitarian entitlements to health care services, health care savings accounts may prove the only feasible and in many cases the most morally justifiable approach. That is, health care savings accounts

1. by protecting private property rights, can sustain an integral element of humans as incarnate persons, an element even more significant than that supported by civil libertarian rights;
2. by protecting private property rights, can sustain a health care financing system that enjoys a moral justification rooted in the property rights of individuals unavailable to health care policy approaches seeking to justify the creation of

    a. democratic voting rights whose scope (i.e., unconstrained through a limited democratic constitutional framework) can lead to the creation of health care entitlements,
    b. democratic voting rights whose scope can lead to egalitarian health care systems.
    These latter require the rational justification of a thick, canonical account of morality that can justify a totalizing political framework, which moral theory and bioethics have failed to supply;

3. by protecting the possibility for responsible individual choice, can nurture an ethos of responsible resources management appropriate to and even essential for decision-making within high-technology societies, which societies often produce high-cost, low-yield interventions.

In a world marked by moral pluralism and irresolvable foundational disagreement, health care savings accounts with their focus on property rights respect individuals as the source of moral authority, while at the same time supporting the integrity of the family in the pursuit of its own vision of resource use and human flourishing.

Health care savings accounts have the consequentialist virtue of supporting the recognition that persons live in families and realize their flourishing in particular moral communities. Such communities can be the source of a particular moral appreciation of virtue and commitment unavailable in a moral framework, which must span a pluralism of moral visions. Such communities can bolster the reliability of relations of trust. Savings accounts also have a morally fungible character that can be recruited to support diverse understandings of moral commitment and moral integrity, which through sustaining the fabric of civil society can sustain a health care system. Once embedded in the practices of particular communities and the commitments of families, family-oriented health care savings accounts can recruit substantive commitments to particular understandings of human flourishing and the substantive appreciation of mutual trust that this can nurture. Even if engaged within a diverse set of understandings of the family and human flourishing, health care savings accounts can support the development of thick understandings of individual and family responsibility. As such, savings accounts can contribute to the moral and symbolic resources of civil society.

Last but not least, health care savings accounts can shape the character of medical markets, in that patients and their families can enter with their own resources rather than with entitlements to care. In this circumstance they will have incentives to be prudent purchasers of health care services and to seek discounted prices individually or in collaboration with others. Because the resources expended at the point of purchase are theirs, they will have good reasons to become responsible participants in a high-technology society. China, by making a commitment to medical savings plans with a family orientation, has the opportunity to help further develop a model that may lead health care policy out of the blind economic and moral alleys that have been pursued in North America and Western Europe.

Notes

1 For a more ample argument regarding the concrete and contextual character of all understandings of beneficence, see Engelhardt (1996, Chaps. 4.3.3 and 4).

2 For an overview of the increase in health care expenditures from 1960 to 1997, see Anderson and Poullier (1999). For an analysis of the distribution of health care expenditures among the American population, see Berc and Monheit (2001). For an overview of the role played by high-technology interventions in American health care in comparison to other countries, see Anderson, Reinhardt, Hussey, and Petrosyan (2002).

3 For discussions of the impact of the growing elderly population on health care costs, and other issues related to health care costs for the elderly, see Miller (2001); Reinhardt (2000); Goldman and Zissimopoulos (2003); Knickman, Hunt, Snell, Alecxih, and Kennell (2003); Morrisey and Jensen (2001); and Lubitz, Greenberg, Gornia, Wartzman, and Gibson (2001).

4 In a Cato Institute study of the economic effects of health care regulation in the United States, Christopher J. Conover reports that "continuation-of-coverage mandates have a net cost of $15.0 billion, while benefit mandates have a net cost of $13.5 billion" (2004, p. 13). In another Cato Institute study, John C. Goodman (2005) discusses some of the problems with proposed national health insurance schemes. See also Barnighausen and Sauerborn (2002).

5 For an overview of the Singapore health care system, see Healthcare Research Group (1999); Duff (2001).

6 The term bioethics was coined by Van Rensselaer Potter (1970a, 1970b, 1971). Potter sought to engender an ethos aimed at preserving the biosphere. "Bioethics" appears to have been either independently coined or fundamentally recast in its meaning by Sargent Shriver and/or André Hellegers (Sargent Shriver, letter to author, January 26, 2001). See also Reich (1994). An overview of the development of bioethics as the new health care morality is provided by Jonsen (1998). For an account of the transformation of medical ethics into bioethics, see Engelhardt (2002).

7 The difficulty in establishing a particular foundation so as to justify a particular moral perspective has been well known for nearly 2000 years. A classical account of these difficulties was provided by Agrippa, a member of the late Academy, who argued that it was impossible to resolve foundational philosophical disputes by sound rational argument. Agrippa took this position because of the centuries-old failure of philosophers to reach a consensus, as well as the circumstance that all argue from within a particular theoretical perspective, rendering competing views to some extent incommensurable. In addition and crucially, philosophical arguments at their foundations inevitably beg the question, argue in a circle, or engage in an infinite regress. Though one might dispute the strength of Agrippa's arguments regarding philosophy in general, the difficulty with regard to moral theory is that a different ranking of values and/or a different ranking of basic moral principles will ground a different morality. Any particular ranking of values and right-making conditions, any particular moral sense, depends on a particular background set of premises and rules of inference necessary to authenticate that ranking, which background premises and rules of inference could have been otherwise. Agrippa's views are recorded by Diogenes Laertius (*Lives of Eminent Philosophers* IX.88) and Sextus Empiricus ("Outlines of Pyrrhonism" I.164). For reflection on these difficulties, see Engelhardt (1996, Chap. 4.3.3).

8 In his influential 1971 account of the theory of justice, it may not appear obvious to the casual reader that Rawls is not in fact establishing a particular moral vision (Rawls, 1971). In his later works this becomes clear, as he takes the position that he is not providing a moral or metaphysical account, but rather an exegesis of the commitments involved in a particular social-democratic constitutional vision (Rawls, 1993). For an example of an account grounded in a reading of John Rawls' *A Theory of Justice* as a moral text, see Daniels (1985).

9 For a more detailed analysis of the inescapably procedural character of any general secular morality, see Engelhardt (1996).

10 Ruiping Fan has made an important contribution to envisaging the power of a contemporary Confucian ethos. See Fan (2002).

11 A remarkable exception to the American health care ideology is the so-call Oregon Plan that was undertaken as a frankly non-egalitarian framework. See Strosberg, Wiener, Baker, and Fein (1992).

12 A good example of how a fervent commitment to health care egalitarianism makes it extremely difficult for societies to move in the direction of health care savings accounts can be taken from recent U.S. Congressional discussions of the matter. For instance, Senator Ted Kennedy, a staunch supporter of moving the U.S. in the direction of a Canadian-style health care system, actually resorted to filibustering his own 1996 health care legislation when health care savings accounts became part of the bill. For a good summary of health care savings accounts and the opposition of this sort that they have encountered, see Scandlen (2001).

13 For an exploration of the cardinal nature of property rights, see Engelhardt (1996, Chap. 4).

[14] From Ruiping Fan I borrowed the phrase "directed fiduciary polity" to describe regimes such as that in Singapore, which is tantamount to a one-party polity and is committed through its embrace of Confucian values to developing secure and economically stable governance, along with a financially sustainable health care system that gives accent to family integrity and autonomy.

References

Anderson, G. F., & Poullier, J. P. (1999, May/June). Health spending, access, and outcomes: Trends in industrialized countries. *Health Affairs, 18*, 178–192.

Anderson, G. F., Reinhardt, U. E., Hussey, P. S., & Petrosyan, V. (2002). It's the prices, stupid: Why the United States is so different from other countries. *Health Affairs, 22*, 89–105.

Barnighausen, T., & Sauerborn, R. (2002). One hundred and eighteen years of the German Health Insurance System: Are there any lessons for middle and low-income countries? *Social Science & Medicine, 54*, 1559–1587.

Berc, M. L., & Monheit, A. C. (2001, March/April). The concentration of health care expenditures, revisited. *Health Affairs, 20*, 9–18.

Conover, C. J. (2004, October 4). Health care regulation: A $169 billion hidden tax. *Policy Analysis*, No. 527.

Daniels, N. (1985). *Just health care*. New York: Cambridge University Press.

Duff, J. (2001). Financing to foster community health care: A comparative analysis of Singapore, Europe, North America and Australia. *Current Sociology, 49*, 135–154.

Engelhardt, H. T., Jr. (1996). *The foundations of bioethics* (2nd ed.). New York: Oxford University Press.

Engelhardt, H. T., Jr. (2002). The ordination of bioethicists as secular moral experts. *Social Philosophy & Policy, 19*, 59–82.

Fan, R. (2002). Reconstructionist Confucianism and health care: An Asian moral account of health care resource allocation. *Journal of Medicine and Philosophy, 27*, 675–684.

Goldman, D. P., & Zissimopoulos, J. M. (2003, May/June). High out-of-pocket health care spending by the elderly. *Health Affairs, 22*, 194–202.

Goodman, J. C. (2005, January 27). Health care in a free society: Rebutting the myths of national health insurance. *Policy Analysis,* No. 532.

Graham, J. (2008). Perils of parallel trade: Reimporting prescription drugs from Canada to the U.S. In H. T. Engelhardt, Jr. & J. R. Garrett (Eds.), *Medical innovation, profit, and bioethics*. Salem, MA: M&M Scrivener Press.

Healthcare Research Group. (1999). *Health services in Singapore: A strategic entry report*. San Diego, CA: Icon Group International.

Jonsen, A. (1998). *The birth of bioethics*. New York: Oxford University Press.

Knickman, J. R., Hunt, K. A., Snell, E. K., Alecxih, L. M. B., & Kennell, D. L. (2003, May/June). Wealth patterns among elderly Americans: Implications for health care affordability. *Health affairs, 22*, 168–173.

Li, B. (2006). Trust is the core of the physician-patient relationship: From the viewpoint of traditional Chinese medical ethics. In J. Tao (Ed.), *China: Bioethics, trust, and the challenge of the market*. New York: Springer.

Lubitz, J., Greenberg, L. G., Gornia, Y., Wartzman, L., & Gibson, D. (2001, March/April). Three decades of health care use by the elderly, 1965–1998. *Health affairs, 20*, 19–32.

Miller, T. (2001, May). Increasing longevity and medicare expenditures. *Demography, 38*, 215–226.

Morrisey, M. A., & Jensen, G. A. (2001, November/December). The near-elderly, early retirees, and managed care. *Health affairs, 20*, 197–206.

National Center for Policy Analysis. (1995, January 9). NCPA health reform plan (W16), excerpted from *Briefing Book on Health Care,* and adapted from Goodman & Musgrave, 1992. Available online at http://www.ncpa.org/w/w16.html. Accessed 06/10/05.

Potter, V. R. (1970a). Bioethics, the science of "survival". *Perspectives in Biology and Medicine, 14*, 127–53.

Potter, V. R. (1970b). Biocybernetics and survival. *Zygon, 5*, 229–46.

Potter, V. R. (1971). *Bioethics, bridge to the future*. Englewood Cliffs, NJ: Prentice-Hall.

Rawls, J. (1971). *A theory of justice*. Cambridge, MA: Harvard University Press.

Rawls, J. (1993). *Political liberalism*. New York: Columbia University Press.

Reich, W. (1994). The word 'bioethics': Its birth and the legacies of those who shaped its meaning. *Kennedy Institute of Ethics Journal, 4*, 319–336.

Reinhardt, U. E. (2000, Spring). Health care for the aging baby boom. *The Journal of Economic Perspectives, 14*, 71–83.

Scandlen, G. (2001, November 2). MSA's can be a windfall for all. *Policy Backgrounder,* No. 157, 1–25. [On-line]. Available at: http://www.ncpa.org/pub/bg/bg157/bg157.pdf. Accessed 07/15/05.

Strosberg, M. A., Wiener, J. M., Baker, R., & Fein, I. A. (Eds.). (1992). *Rationing America's medical care: The Oregon plan and beyond.* Brookings Dialogues on Public Policy. Washington, DC: The Brookings Institution.

Part III
Trust, Profit, Scarcity, and Integrity: Confucian Thought and Traditional Morality

Confucian Trust, Market and Health Care Reform

Julia Tao

Health care systems in the world are beset by a common problem. The problem to frame a moral basis for health care policy that provides all citizens with basic coverage, encourages innovation, contains costs, and supports commitment to trust and responsibility which can guarantee the reliable function of the market and the ethical behaviour of health care professionals.

This paper begins with the background recognition that, first, while medical advances offer the prospect of lowering morbidity and morality risks through the development of ever more effective health care interventions, they at the same time generate more costs, particularly in societies with an increasing proportion of the population advancing beyond retirement age. Second, there are evidences that an egalitarian health care system which provides all citizens with all health care services can create moral hazards by removing incentives for the prudent choice and use of health care resources. Third, market forces can contribute to the efficient distribution of medical goods and services, and to spur medical innovation in a medical market, if an appropriate balance is achieved between the roles of the government, private investment, and the market. Fourth, the paper points out that creating a market in China would need to proceed with extreme care and caution since in our study, there are also serious problems with the move towards the marketization of health care which threatening to erode trust and to undermine care in the Chinese health system. While liberalizing the health market can be useful for creating dynamism and diversity in the system, strengthening public health care to protect equity and accessibility in the face of huge economic inequality in China under transition to the market economy will be essential.

The intention of this paper is to examine the possible contribution of Confucian cultural and moral resources to guide the development of a responsible market context for the private provision of health care which can sustain commitments of trust and reliability. It begins by examining the concept of trust and identifies three levels of trust: *first-order trust, second-order trust*, and *third-order trust*, which are pertinent as the basis of freedom, autonomy and responsibility in modern

J. Tao, Ph.D.
Department of Public and Social Administration, City University of Hong Kong
e-mail: sajulia@cityu.edu.hk

J. Tao (ed.), *China: Bioethics, Trust, and the Challenge of the Market*,
© Springer Science+Business Media B.V. 2008

governance. It analyses the relevance of these three levels of trust for the nurturance of a responsible market context for the development of a private sector in health care. It concludes by examining the Confucian account of trust in the Chinese moral tradition and argues how it might contribute to a re-visioning of the ideal of trust to embrace the three levels of trust for the development of a responsible market in private health care within the context of a robust public sector in China.

1 Trust in Health Care – Where Are We Now?

A study was conducted in both the public and the private hospitals in Shandong in 2004 to understand how recent developments in health care reform have influenced the doctor–patient relationship and affected trust in medical practice in general. Data were gathered through face to face in-depth interviews with health care professionals, hospital administrators, government health department officials, nurses, patients, patients' family members, and representatives of the pharmaceutical industry. The interviews yielded immensely rich and interesting data. There is a clear division of opinions regarding the transition to a market economy and the impact of market forces on health care reform in China. The division represents a slit between, on the one hand, those who see market forces and market values as destructive of trust and professional integrity; and those, on the other hand, who welcome market freedom and market competition because they can enhance trust in the profession.

1.1 Market Forces Erode Trust

Those who consider market to be eroding trust cite the following negative features of the current health care system to argue that doctors no longer act in the best interest of their patients; that the medical profession is on the whole self-serving, irresponsible and uncaring. They are concerned about the following phenomena in the health care sector because they undermine trust:

- Red Packet Phenomenon – distrust of doctors
- Hospital Deposit System – no money, no treatment culture
- Prevalent practice of Kick-Back – personal gain and profit
- Over Prescription of drugs – neglect of patients' interests
- Dishonest Practice Promotion – deception and dishonesty
- Delayed Discharge of Patients – increase of personal income
- Substandard Professional Competency – no incentive for self-improvement
- Defensive Medicine – concern about self-protection

The following are some direct quotes from the respondents regarding their views on the negative aspects of introducing a market in health care in China:

1. On the Erosion of Trust in Doctor–Patient Relationship
   "Doctors' concern for economic benefits has made them trust-worthless"

"Since most patients are usually ignorant of the state of their illnesses and diseases, they could only listen to the advice of doctors."

2. On the Red Packet Phenomenon
"... some patients give 'red pockets' [紅包] to doctors because they are worried that the doctors would not carry out their duties faithfully if they do not give them 'red pocket'."
"It does happen pretty often. It happens more often in large hospitals because 'red pocket' is more necessary since there are more serious illnesses being dealt with in large hospitals."
"The root for the rise of 'red pocket' is distrust between individuals. It is mainly patients' distrust of doctors."
3. On the Hospital Deposit System
"For peasants, they would be allowed to stay in hospital for a $500 deposit [押金]. However, their drugs would be terminated if the deposit is used up."
"For 'government-subsidized' patients, they would be requested to pay $5000 or $10000 when they in fact their treatment cost might only be $2000; and patients would not be allowed to leave the hospital even if they have recovered, until they have exhausted their deposit."
4. On the Kick-Back Culture
"A key concern is that the large sum of 'kick-back' [回扣] taken by doctors and hospitals in the purchase of medical equipments is transferred into medical fees to be paid by patients."
"For example, one of my friends produced a large-scale CT-machine. The initial price was $4 million, while the final price was $6 million. The difference, $2 million, was taken as 'kick-back' by a hospital head and those in the relevant department of the hospital."
"A lot of doctors would take advantage of 'kick-back' from drugs sellers as a kind of 'extra income'. There are direct linkages between doctors and drugs sellers.
5. On Over-Prescription of Drugs
"... 99% of doctors would simply consider their own interests. For example, they prescribed a lot of drugs for patients. If drugs of $10 would be enough to treat a patient, they would prescribe drugs of $30."
"It is very common that the amount of drugs prescribed to a patient is a multiple of the amount of drugs that the patient really needs."
6. On Dishonest Practice Promotion
"Up to 95% of medical advertisements are false or illegal."
"Medical advertisements are examined by the Health Administration Department [衛生行政部門], but managed by the Business and Industrial Administration Department [工商行政部門] which has the authority to punish illegal advertising; but law enforcement is poor and ineffective."
7. On Excessive Treatment
"The 'body-check' for my father has been repeated three times."
In addition, medical equipments is also a source from which doctors could make "extra income".

8. On the Corruption of Professional Integrity
   "Those small hospitals always lie; they cannot provide real quality services."
   "Doctors of the 1980s were really nice. The relationships were very good and simple."
   "To the doctors of the 1980s, the health of patients always comes first."
   "The central value of market economy is competition. People are more money-minded, pragmatic and materialistic as a result. Moreover, people are individualistic and human relationships are based on materials."

Regarding the positive aspects of introducing a market in health care in China, some of the respondents made the following observations:

1. On the Establishment of a Patient-centred Ethos
   "The only way out for private hospital is to improve the job attitudes of the staff."
   "We are trying to explore medical services that are not provided by 'large hospitals' such as treatments of chronic diseases."
   "Doctors are very nice to the patients. Our hospital has its emphasis on 'customer-oriented' attitudes towards patients."
2. On the Promotion of an Accountability Culture
   "The 'daily information update' [一日一清單] is displayed in hospitals, available to patients and the public. It provides all information regarding the charges of medical treatments."
3. On the Promotion of Rational Choice and Responsibility among Patients
   "Patients who have come to our hospital are rational. Some of them had compared our hospital with other large hospitals of the province such as the [省立醫院，齊魯醫院] (Provincial hospitals) in terms of the prices and effectiveness of medical treatments before they came to our hospital."
   "Patients of our hospital would often make comparisons and chose carefully."
   "Yes. They would deliberate on their decisions thoroughly."
4. On the Creation of Incentives for Innovations
   "First, we try to enhance the quality and effectiveness of our medical services in order to win the confidence and trust of patients."
   "Private hospitals need to develop specializations in order to compete and survive."
   "Second, we explore new medical services and experiment with new drugs."
5. On the Empowerment of Patients
   In "large hospitals", patients tend to believe that they are "begging" for medical services. Therefore, they would not speak out even if they had been treated badly. In our hospitals, patients have a stronger sense of "autonomy" and "equality".

1.2 Market Competition Enhances Trust

But there is also another group of respondents who welcome a private market in health care. They are of the view that a private market can bring in competition, encourage more rational use of resources, more innovation, greater cost-effectiveness, more trust and better relationship between doctors and patients. They argue that under market conditions, they have to seek continuous self-improvement by constantly paying attention to promote:

- Patient-oriented Service Ethos
- Reliability and Accountability Culture
- Accessibility and Freedom of Information
- Efficiency in the distribution of health care goods and resources
- Autonomy and rational choice among patients
- Evidence-based medicine and cost-effectiveness in decision making
- Performance-based Reward System
- Incentive for innovations
- Patient autonomy and personal responsibility

2 Making Sense of the Confusion About Trust

The picture which has emerged seems to be highly confusing. Has there been a loss in trust, a decline in trust, or a de-emphasis on trust in the health care enterprise as a consequence of the health care reform in China? Or has there been a strengthening of trust because of the emergence of a private market in medicine in the form of private hospitals? I would say that the answer is both 'yes' and 'no' depending on which concept of trust we are referring to.

Discussions about trust in the healthcare system can in fact be concerned with three different levels or orders of trust: 'paternalistic' trust, 'strategic' trust and 'moralistic' trust. But most discussions tend to focus on either 'paternalistic' trust or 'startegic' trust. They are sometimes referred to as 'first-order' trust and 'second-order' trust. But I want to draw attention to a third level of trust, which can be termed 'moralistic' trust. This is the third order of trust. I shall argue that this 'moralistic' aspect or level of trust is even more foundational and essential than the other two levels, although it is often the first two levels of trust that seem to be at the centre of public debate. Heath Care reform can impact on all three levels of trust. Likewise, all three levels of trust are necessary for a robust and reliable health care system.

To the question whether we have a problem of trust in our health care system, my short answer would be there is no doubt that there has been a certain loss, decline and de-emphasis on the first-order trust, namely 'paternalistic' trust; but there is also a corresponding rise, increase and emphasis on second-order trust, namely 'strategic' trust. Importantly also, what seems to be happening is an emerging shift in the moral foundation of the medical enterprise itself, that is in the third-level trust, namely 'moralistic' trust. There are indications that this third level of trust in medicine is seriously under threat; it would need to be strengthened and re-emphasized if the moral character of medicine is to be preserved.

3 First Order Trust: Paternalistic Trust

3.1 Paternalistic Trust: The Personal Dimension of Trust

Paternalistic Trust is the basis of the traditional medical ethics, both in the west and the east. It is grounded in the unequal status and unequal power relationship between doctors and patients. The doctor patient relationship is recognized as a paternal relationship because of patients' vulnerability and need for protection for their well being. The direction of responsibility is always from those with higher status, greater authority and more resources towards those who have less. In return they are reciprocated with the trust of those who are supposed to benefit from their status, authority and resources.

We can find the common ideal of paternalistic trust enshrined in the Hippocratic Oath in the west and also upheld as a moral imperative in the first Chinese classic book of traditional medicine, the *Huangdi neigjing* ('The Emperors Interior Scripture') which appeared during the 'Warring States' period (475–221 BC). Under this moral imperative, doctors are committed to use their knowledge to fulfill the duties of saving lives and relieving suffering, offering treatment to patients with equal respect regardless of their social status or their means. They are always to act in the best interests of the patients who are under their care.

The ideal of paternalistic trust is dependent on the benevolent disposition of the doctors. It emphasizes the moral character and integrity of doctors. The problem with paternalistic trust is that it may give too much power and too much responsibility to the medical professionals, creating dependence, encouraging inefficiency, moral hazards, lack of patient autonomy, and abuse of trust.

4 Second Order Trust: Strategic Trust

4.1 Strategic Trust: The Procedural Dimension of Trust

Strategic trust locates trust in institutions and procedures instead of in actors and persons. It is a way of compensating distrust in persons with trust in institutions. It is characterized by the development of the rule of law, accountability systems, checks and balances, rules, laws and procedures to protect individual rights, freedom and autonomy.

The emergence of strategic trust marks a level of higher abstraction, from personal to procedural trust, from trust in persons to trust in abstract rules and impersonal laws. It provides a kind of backup or insurance for those who would be ready to risk trust, a disincentive for those who would contemplate breaches of trust, or a corrective of actual violation of trust, if they occur. It is also spurred by the development in favour of an understanding of human flourishing in terms of a kind of autonomous individualism rather than in terms of the cultivation of traditional virtues and the development of moral character. Central to autonomous individualism is the presumption that persons are self-interested rational individuals who are committed to self determination and advancement of their individual interests. Choice, autonomy, individual rights and self-responsibility are the core values of autonomous individualism. For example, the presumption in favour of treating patients as autonomous individuals has led to the development, among many other things, of informed consent as an institution in modern medicine to strengthen trust in the doctor–patient relationship.

Instead of emphasizing that 'it is in one's duty to be trustworthy', which is the central tenet of paternalistic trust, strategic trust emphasizes that 'it is in one's interest to be trustworthy.' Instead of assuming that we are all altruistic and benevolent human beings, the starting point of strategic trust is that we are all self-interested and self-serving individuals; doctors and politicians are no exception.

Since human beings are self-interested and are rightly so, they can be trusted to use their special advantages for the good of others only if they are convinced that it will be in their own self-interest to do so, that it pays to be trusted or that it hurts to be found not trustworthy. On this account, trust does not depend on the trustworthiness of a person.

Strategic trust emphasizes the instrumental or strategic reasons why one should trust another. On this account, trust itself has no moral content. Trust is a matter of mere rational expectations about the behaviour of others. It is grounded in the truster's assessment of the trusted's interest in fulfilling the trust. In other words, my trust in you is typically encapsulated in your interest in fulfilling my trust. Russell Hardin (1998) describes this understanding of trust as 'encapsulated interest'.

The basic assumption is that the law itself is sufficient to guarantee social cooperation among self-directed individuals motivated entirely by incentives of self-interest. Obedience to the law can be motivated by compelling incentives of self-interest even when there is no trust. The important insights of Hardin's strategic account of trust is to draw attention to the fact that trust is risky, that trust has a cost and that it is not always warranted. In drawing attention to the risks and vulnerabilities in trust, he reminds us that trust is a function of the rational monitoring of risks by individuals. Relationships of trust are no more than mere expectations grounded in the interests of the trusted to fulfill the trust. Trust is largely a matter of rational probabilistic expectation.

Critics of strategic trust have objected that it is too impoverished as an account of trust to be able to provide the basis for a robust civil society and an active citizenry who are mutually committed to taking collective action to achieve autonomy and self-government. Institutional mechanisms are designed to control distrust. They are driven by the purpose to institutionalize distrust in order to protect expectation and to support the practice of probabilistic expectation. They cannot be a source of trust.

In fact it has been argued that the pursuit of ever more perfect accountability provides citizens and consumers, patients and parents in modern society with more information, more comparisons, more complaints systems; but it also builds a culture of suspicion, low morale, professional cynicism which ultimately undermine rather than support trust. Ultimately, this can lead to what Michael Power (1994) has called the 'audit explosion.'

It is of equal importance that it is not only distrust but also trust that is institutionally grounded and has to be institutionally implemented. As Onora O'Neill (2002) has pointed out, good governance is possible only if institutions and professionals are allowed some margin for autonomy and self-governance of a form appropriate to their particular tasks. What this means in essence is that to be pervasive and lasting, trust cannot be merely due to efficient control. How to keep the balance between the institutionalized distrust on the one hand and a minimal level of trust by the citizens on the other continues to be an important question for social life and for political systems. soul-searching question.

Perhaps the major weakness of Hardin's account of strategic trust is that he fails to see trust as a moral good. It is a functional prerequisite, or an essential condition of all autonomous communities. Both the rule of law and the free market depend on trust. Trust is the basis of freedom, autonomy and responsibility. It is a bottom-up resource complementary to top down authority. In the west, John Locke [1690] (1988) has shown that it is especially a constitutional government with responsibility towards its citizen that is based on the principle of trust. It is founded on the trust of the citizens in that the government would only exercise power in order to protect each citizen's property, namely their life, liberty, and estate (Locke TGII #123). Claus Offe has also pointed out that trust as well solidarity are necessary prerequisites for any democratic authority (1999:42).

5 Third Order Trust: Moralistic Trust

5.1 Moralistic Trust: The Symbolic Dimension of Trust

This brings us to the concept of moralistic trust. Moralistic trust recognizes trust as a moral good. Moralistic trust is essential to sustaining a culture of trust in the community. Cooperation is possible only if there exists a minimal standard of mutual trust that no one gets cheated or betrayed. According to Uslander (2002), moralistic trust is not about having faith in particular people or even groups of people. This is trust in people whom we don't know and who are likely to be different from ourselves. It is a general outlook on human nature and is an essential foundation of a civil society.

Moralistic trust expresses the belief that others share your fundamental moral values and therefore should be treated as you would wish to be treated by them. The value they share may vary from person to person. What matters is a sense of connection with others because you see them as members of your community whose interest must be taken seriously. Moralistic trust is a commandment to treat people *as if* they were trustworthy. Moralistic trust is what binds people together.

Moralistic trust is based on the assumption that the human subject is someone whose behaviours are driven not only just by the desire to seek and advance his/her individual self-interest, but more importantly perhaps, also driven by a shared commitment and benevolence towards others.

Moralistic trust provides the rationale for getting involved with other people and working toward compromises. It connects us to people who are different from ourselves, not merely to people we already know or folks just like us. Trusting strangers means accepting them into our 'moral community.' Strangers may look different from us, they may have different ideologies or religions. But we believe that there is an underlying commonality of values. We have obligations to one another. We take others' moral claims seriously.

Moralistic trust, as third-order trust, also draws attention to the symbolic aspect of trust. Moralistic trust becomes effective by giving a visible expression to the basic common values of the citizens. Such basic common values can only be expressed by institutions in a *symbolic* way. Society need to make its basic stock of commonly shared values visible in its key institutions. They are the motivational triggers in a way that actualize trust over and over again. Normative integration of society is successful only if there is a basic stock of common values and if the symbolic expression of common values can support mutual commitment and shared responsibility in the form of some common enterprise or common good.

A public health care system which guarantees a basic level of medical care to all those in need is an embodiment of trust as mutual commitment and mutual responsibility in the symbolic sense. What gives a common good a special sort of value distinctive from the functional value of other kinds of good is the *commonness* that constitutes its value, the value of the good. Societies can become destabilized if the elementary resources of trust are exhausted, or if its common goods are no longer symbolic expressions of common values.

A robust society where human rights are protected, citizens are autonomous, markets are reliable and welfare are promoted requires the flourishing of all three orders of trust: paternalistic trust, strategic and moralistic trust.

6 Confucian Trust: Paternalistic, Strategic or Moralistic?

When Confucius was asked about government by his disciple, Tzu-kung, more than 2000 years ago, he said that three things are needed for government: weapons, food and trust. If a ruler can't hold on to all three, he should give up the weapons first and the food next. Trust should be guarded to the end: without trust we cannot stand (*Analects* 12:7).

Trust is an important value in Confucian philosophy. It has supported a long tradition of paternalistic trust in the Chinese history. As a political virtue, trust is grounded in the duty of government agents to serve the interests of citizens. Confucius himself had reminded those in government that: 'In guiding a state of a thousand chariots, approach your duties with reverence and be trustworthy in what you say; avoid excesses in expenditure and love your fellow men; employ the labour of the common people only in the right seasons' (*Analects* 1:5).

To a certain extent, this interpretation is similar to the view of Locke, who had also argued that the justification of trust lies in those agents 'whom society hath set over it self, with this express or tacit Trust, that it shall be imployed for their good, and the preservation of their Property' (171:381).

Trust is an important value in Confucian philosophy because of its moral ideal of ren. *Ren* is translated as humanity, love or benevolence. Such a moral ideal identifies a good government as one that serves the best interests of the people. But Confucian *ren* is more than benevolence of the government in providing for the welfare of the people in return for submission and compliance. A virtuous ruler who practices benevolent government must also take the realization of the virtuous life of the people as the highest goal. But a good government should first be characterized by a virtuous rule, because only those who are virtuous can win the hearts of the people. Rulers must actively cultivate themselves in order to refine their virtues and characters.

It is therefore not surprising that on numerous occasions, both Confucius as well as Mencius have emphasized the importance of the duty of government to provide for food and to provide security from war which are the necessary conditions for the general populace to obey the law, to honour obligations and to uphold trust. Confucian understanding of the conditions of trust are in this sense very different from those defined earlier by Hardin. As Mencius observed:

> . . . a wise ruler will decide on such a plan for the people's means of support as to make sure that they can support their parents as well as their wives and children, and that they have enough food in good years, and are saved from starvation in bad (*Mencius* 1A:16).

He firmly believed that

> This is the way of the common people. Those with constant means of support will have constant hearts, while those without constant means will not have constant hearts. Lacking constant hearts, they will go astray and get into excesses, stopping at nothing. To punish them after they have fallen foul of the law is to set a trap for the people (3A:3).

Furthermore, benevolent government requires more than the mere provision for basic needs and the lending of help to the people, benevolent government also demands the practice of equitable distribution of resources, clear allocation of benefits and adequate protection of interests as Mencius had further observed that:

> Benevolent government must begin with land demarcation. When boundaries are not properly drawn, the division of land according to the well-field system and the yield of grain used for paying officials cannot be equitable.... Once the boundaries are correctly fixed, there will be no difficulty in settling the distribution of land and the determination of emoulment (ibid).

Drawing on the moral principle of extension, Mencius, more than 2000 years ago, articulated a vision of how institutions of the state can serve to harmonize the relationship between private interest and the common good, when he put forward a proposal for the *ching*-field system, commonly translated as the 'well-field' system. It is a system which divides a piece of land into nine plots. When a piece of land is divided into nine plots, it looks like the Chinese character '*ching*' (井) for a 'well'. Hence, the system is known as *ching*-field.

> If those who own land within each *ching* befriend one another both at home and abroad, help each other to keep watch, and succor each other in illness, they will live in love and harmony. A *ching* is a piece of land measure one *li* square, and each *ching* consists of 900 *mu*. Of these the central plot of 100 *mu* belongs to the state, while the other eight plots of 100 *mu* each are held by eight families who share the duty of caring for the plot owned by the state. Only when they have done this duty dare they turn to their own affairs (*Mencius* 3A:3).

Mencius' 'well-field system' tells a story of supporting the common good while cultivating one's private interest. It instantiates a much broader symbolic meaning of a non-individualistic self-understanding of the human subject which is relational in its perspective and communal in its orientation, being committed to both cultivating one's own private interests and to the broader concerns of sustaining the common good beyond what lies beyond one's immediate, private interest. It shows how institutions can support altruism for the nurturance of trust and reciprocity in the community while at the same time generating food and sustenance for the satisfaction of human needs and interests.

Thus we can see that in Confucian moral tradition, trust is also valued as a moral good rather than as a mere strategy in social life. Neither is it valued for its paternalistic function alone. It is an expression of a commitment to a vision of common humanity, which imposes a moral duty of benevolent regard as a way of showing respect for the dignity and humanity in the other person.

Confucius himself had said that he had three goals in life: Respect for the old, Care for the young, and Trust between friends (*Analects* 5:26). Trust is important not only just as a political virtue for government, it is also an essential element of the Confucian conception of the good life.

As pointed out earlier, the Confucian account of trust is the expression of the moral ideal of *ren*. Confucian emphasis on the inner life of the moral agent as the basis of morality can also lend support to the claim that the sources of moralistic trust lies in our culture and disposition. In this way, it can provide a healthy counterbalance to the over-reliance on institutions and on the over-emphasis of distrust of all authority which are major causes for the erosion of a culture of trust in democracy. It draws attention to the importance of self-cultivation for the building of trust and for sustaining a culture of trust instead of adopting a deceptively simple and easy way out of the structural scarcity of trust.

What is clear from the Confucian perspective is that the way out of the dilemma of trust will have to be negotiated through embracing a different perspective on the fundamental nature of the human agent, a different approach to ground the moral foundation of trust, and a different model of civil society underpinned by strong civic virtues.

From the Confucian ethical perspective, human beings are distinguished from other species by their potential for moral virtues. Morality rather than rationality or self-determination is emphasized as the distinguishing characteristics of humanity. The source of human dignity also lies in our potential for moral virtues and for developing our moral character. According to Mencius's thesis of human nature, (one of the founders of the Confucian moral tradition), human beings are born with four seeds or four potentials of moral virtues: *Ren*, *yi*, *li*, and *zhi* . They are also the 'four beginnings' or 'four moral possibilities' of the virtues of benevolence, humaneness, righteousness, propriety and wisdom (*Mencius* 2A:6). When fully developed, these four seeds become the mind of compassion, the mind of shame, the mind of modesty and the mind of right and wrong. Among these four virtues, *ren* is the highest virtue.

These moral potentials constitute the source of human dignity and our common humanity. Trust is an important value because it is the quality of being reliable. To be reliable is to respect the humanity and the human dignity in the other person and to take them seriously. When Confucius replied to his disciple that no government can stand when trust is lost, he was referring to moralistic trust. The loss of trust in this sense implies the loss of commitment to a vision of common humanity, loss of a common bond which connects the individual with the collective, and loss of a common morality which harmonizes the private good with the common good. Should there be a deficit in arms, the state may survive, even if there is deficit in food, the state is still likely to survive, but when there is a deficit in moralistic trust, the state will become collapse and become ungovernable.

Confucian account of trust emphasizes paternalistic trust, procedural trust and moralistic trust, with moralistic as foundational to the other notions of trust. Moralistic trust is not something one can generate from rules and institutions, nor is it something one can buy or sell in the market. Neither can it be called into existence by command of authority. It is we need to preserve the trust in our public health care system and not undermine it at the same time, because trust is a key ingredient of the possibility of a common vision for any society trying to uphold freedom, autonomy, responsibility and self-rule among its members.

In a country like China, in particular, where such huge disparities exist between the rich and the poor, between the cities and the villages, we need a robust sense of civic citizenship to underpin autonomy and responsibility, which is not just based upon non-interference, mutual tolerance or the free pursuance of private interests. We need mutual engagement and mutual concern based on a vision of common humanity beyond strategic trust as emphasized in the Confucian vision of trust, to remind us of our shared fate and mutual responsibility, both at the local level as well as at the global level.

Such a vision of trust is essential to the robust development of medicine which is a common good and an expression of symbolic trust in our society. Moralistic trust is not only essential to the practice of medicine. It is in fact the essence of medicine. It is constitutive of medicine as a humanistic profession itself. There can be no medicine in the absence of this ideal of trust. Medicine as a common good is an expression of symbolic trust and the embodiment of our mutual trust and commitment to our common humanity. In our attempts to regenerate our public health care system and in our efforts to develop a reliable private medicine in China, one should never lose sight of the Confucian insight that the foundation of trust is morality. Nor should one forget that trust cannot be merely due to efficient control or strategic calculations.

References

Hardin, R. (1998). Trust in government. In V. Braithwaite & M. Levi (Eds.), *Trust and governance.* New York: Russell Sage Foundation.

Lau, D. C. (Trans.). (1970). *Mencius.* Penguin Books.

Lau, D. C. (Trans.). (1972). *Analects.* The Chinese University of Hong Kong.

Locke, J. [1690] (1988). *Two treatises of government.* In P. Laslett (Ed.). Cambridge: Cambridge University Press.

Offe, C. (1996). Social capital: Concepts and hypotheses. *American Journal of Political Science, 24,* 633–51.

Offe, C. (1999). How can we trust our fellow citizens? In M. Warren (Ed.), *Democracy and trust.* Cambridge: Cambridge University Press.

O'Neill, O. (2002). *A question of trust.* Cambridge: Cambridge University Press.

Power, M. (1994). *The audit explosion.* London: Demos.

Uslaner, E. M. (2002). *The moral foundations of trust.* Cambridge: Cambridge University Press.

The Pursuit of an Efficient, Sustainable Health Care System in China

The Role of Health Care Organizations[1]

Ana Iltis

1 Introduction

Chinese social and political institutions are evolving as the Chinese economy becomes increasingly market oriented. Policy makers in China have the opportunity to learn from their own past as well as from the experiences of other nations as they reform particular policies, institutions, and social structures. One major area of consideration as China moves forward is its health care system. All nations make decisions that shape health care delivery, whether the government pays for and delivers all health care, the government plays no role in paying for or delivering health care, or there is a mixed public/private system. Thus, reforming the Chinese health care system is among the important tasks facing Chinese policy makers.

The key players in a health care system include patients, health care professionals, and health care organizations. In some systems, independent third-party payers may also play a key role in the system. In reforming their health care system, the Chinese will make decisions concerning the relationship among these participants and the particular roles that are to be played by each. Among other choices, decisions will be made about:

1. Who is permitted to provide health care and under what circumstances health care services may be rendered. For example, will health care professionals be licensed by the state? What will be the scope of such licenses, e.g., will physicians be permitted to sell pharmaceutical products or will physicians write prescriptions that must be filled by another party?
2. Who will pay for health care.
3. Who may own or operate health care organizations.
4. How the costs of health care services will be determined.
5. What rules and regulations health care providers will be obligated to follow and what the consequences will be for breaches of law or policy.

A. Iltis, Ph.D.
Center for Health Care Ethics, Saint Louis University, Saint Louis, Missouri, USA
e-mail: iltisas@slu.edu

J. Tao (ed.), *China: Bioethics, Trust, and the Challenge of the Market*,

© Springer Science+Business Media B.V. 2008

This paper focuses on one of the key players in a health care delivery system – health care organizations – and explores the role such organizations can play as China reforms its health care system. It is imperative that we examine the types of health care organizations a particular health care system can and should accommodate because health care organizations, and not merely individual physicians, nurses, and other health care professionals, shape the delivery of health care. We also must examine the concerns generated by the existence of diverse health care organizations. In this paper, I (1) demonstrate that it is reasonable and prudent to allow for the existence of different types of health care organizations in a society; (2) discuss the importance of those institutions maintaining their integrity; (3) explain what it is for institutions to maintain their integrity; (4) identify some of the reasons it can be difficult to maintain diversity among health care organizations; and (5) identify some important ways to resolve conflicts that arise when different types of organizations co-exist in a society. I argue that the existence of different types of health care organizations is sufficiently important that health care systems, social policies, and laws should not only permit but encourage diversity and integrity.

An essential element of supporting organizational integrity in health care is creating a market within which diverse organizations can fulfill the needs and interests of different individuals and groups. Although discussions of markets sometimes treat the market as an enemy of integrity or even of decent behavior, the opposite is true. Markets hold those who offer and buy goods and services accountable. In doing so, markets encourage responsibility and fidelity to promises and commitments and discourage fraud and corruption. Those who make promises and fail to keep them are punished in the market place. Customers will not return and customers will share with others their negative experience. For example, if patients find that they have been charged for services they did not receive or have been prescribed unnecessary treatments in a health care organization, they may not return and they may encourage others to seek care elsewhere. The health care organization will suffer a decline in its patient base and, ultimately, its income. A health care market in which patients can choose among providers may alleviate the present-day practice in China by which physicians sometimes prescribe medications patients do not need or prescribe more expensive medications than patients need so that they may profit from the sale of pharmaceuticals. Properly employed, markets also provide a means for maintaining moral, cultural, and religious traditions. Persons who are steeped in a tradition may demand, for example, that their health care environment respect their tradition or culture. Health care organizations that fail to do so will "lose" their patients; patients will go elsewhere for their care. Individuals and groups may treat the failure to respect tradition as grounds for abandoning an organization in favor of another. In a market environment, organizations that fail to maintain their integrity will be punished. Because, as I demonstrate in this paper, it is of great importance that organizations do maintain their integrity, the incentives and accountability offered by the market that promote integrity should be recognized and utilized.

2 Organizational Diversity: Public and Private

To appreciate the importance and potential diversity in a health care marketplace, imagine four different types of health care organizations.

1. Health Maintenance Organization (HMO): Patients have restricted access to physicians, hospitals, and tests; all care must be obtained from physicians within the organization and all visits to specialists must be approved by a patient's primary physician; limited coverage is available for expensive treatments such as organ transplants; interventions meant to enhance lifestyle but not cure illness – such as wigs for persons who have lost their hair from alopecia or chemotherapy – are not covered; emergency treatment is covered; patients pay very low premiums. An HMO may be operated by a not-for-profit or charitable organization that seeks to expand access to health care. An HMO also might be operated by a for-profit company.

2. Boutique Care/Concierge Care/Retainer Medicine: Patients pay high premiums or individual fee-for-service rates; typically they have access to their physician 24 hours/day often including cell phone and email access; and they are guaranteed short waiting times.[2] Boutique Care also might include staying in a hospital or an area of a hospital designed to provide patients with luxuries, comforts and conveniences not available in most hospital settings. Many physicians and organizations that offer these services do not accept insurance payments.

3. Public Hospital or Clinic: The organization is supported through taxation and private donations; health care often is provided by physicians and nurses in training who are supervised by licensed providers; a wide range of services is available – in part because trainees need exposure to many different types of treatments; waiting rooms often are crowded and wait times may be lengthy; treatment generally is free to patients or provided for very low fees.

4. Religious or Belief-Based Hospital: The organization has specific commitments about how health care will be provided and which services are offered. In the United States the most common faith-based health care organization are Roman Catholic hospitals. Such hospitals are owned and operated by a variety of groups, but all are expected to follow basic guidelines for providing health care in a Catholic context.[3] Other religious groups also have hospitals. For example, Loma Linda University Medical Center is a Seventh-Day Adventist institution that adheres to basic dietary restrictions followed by the church.[4] One can imagine other belief-based organizations built not around religious commitments but on some other cultural or traditional commitment, such as a commitment to the centrality of the family.

Patients and health care professionals in these four types of organizations would have very different experiences because of the nature of each organization. Moreover, to maintain its integrity, each organization may have to act in quite different ways. These differences are important, I will argue, for meeting the health care needs and interests of a diverse population.

3 It is Reasonable and Prudent to Encourage the Existence of Various Types of Health Care Organizations in Society

There are four principal reasons for which it is reasonable and prudent to encourage the existence of diverse types of health care organizations in a society. I suggest that it also is reasonable to establish some limits, or side-constraints, on the types of organizations that may be permitted to exist. Later I argue that it is important for health care organizations to maintain their moral integrity to preserve the benefits of having a diverse system. I consider here the benefits of such diversity.

Reason 1: Diversity reduces burdens on the government system. In health systems in which individuals have access only to government-run and funded health care, the government must bear the burden of all health care. Some individuals may opt out of the system altogether and receive health care in other countries, relieving the state-funded system. For example, some Canadian patients who have chosen to leave Canada to come to the United States to pay for health care to receive services not available in Canada or to avoid waiting for treatment.[5] But generally a system that is operated and funded solely by the government will bear the health care responsibilities of all those eligible to use the system. Once alternatives are available, some individuals will choose to opt out of that system for some other choice. That decision may be based on some principled belief or conviction, such as a desire to receive health care in an environment that promotes particular values. Others will choose alternatives for convenience or because they believe the quality of care to be superior. Those persons no longer will be a burden on the government system, or will be less of a burden on that system.

Reason 2: Diversity, competition, and the potential for profit promote efficiency, innovation, and technological progress. Where there is competition and the opportunity for profit, there is motivation to develop new technologies, pharmaceutical products, medical devices, and procedures. Initially newly developed technologies, drugs, devices, and procedures may be expensive and available only to those willing and able to pay more for them. But they may eventually be available for less, or they may turn out to be cost effective. That is, they may save money in the long-run. These savings may be savings to the health system per se: a new treatment may be less expensive than older options. They also may be savings to society because, for example, patients may lose less time from work. Long-term, individuals and society may be more productive and will spend less money on health care. But if no one in a society, whether an individual or a company, stands to make money from developing new devices and drugs, there may be little motivation to do so. Moreover, until new medications or devices are shown to be cost effective, public and private insurers may be unwilling to pay for them. Only those willing and able to pay themselves may have access to new pharmaceuticals and medical devices for some time.

For organizations that are concerned with profit, there is greater motivation to reduce costs by saving money through improved efficiency and a reduction in errors. Consider the use of computerized medication delivery systems in hospitals. A number of hospitals in the United States now have computer software that enables nurses and physicians to confirm that they are giving the right does of medication to the right patient at the right time and that the medication is not contra-indicated by anything else the patient is taking or any scheduled procedure. Such systems are expensive, but they have been shown to significantly reduce medication errors. Such errors cost money, time, and lives. Thus such systems may be cost-effective and may improve patient care and satisfaction. Unless an organization has a clear motivation to improve care, decrease long-term costs, or reduce errors, there is no incentive for anyone to develop such a product or for any particular organization to invest in it. Private health care organizations may have a greater incentive, in some cases, to invest in the development of new technology. In the long run, such investment may benefit society overall even if in the short-term it benefits only those who can afford it.[6]

Diversity in a health system creates room for competition and profit, conditions necessary for innovation. In a diverse system, such innovation may benefit few people initially, and some may never have direct access to the benefits. But as time passes, the benefits of innovation typically accrue to more and more people.[7] Moreover, if a society were to require immediate equal access to all new health care products, devices, and services, it would be too costly to encourage or even permit innovation. The costs of equal access would be too great.

Reason 3: Systems that disallow diversity and require equality must provide uniformly low levels of care. Requiring equality in a health care system means that one must set a uniformly low level of care for all. Providing a uniformly high level of care will render the system unsustainable. Insofar as Chinese policy makers seek to avoid these extremes in the new Chinese health care system, the important role of diverse health care organizations should be recognized. Although the United States' system is not a single system with a uniformly equal level of care available to all, consider the following points as (1) evidence of a system that is trying to promote equality and (2) evidence that such attempts can have negative consequences and be unsustainable.

EMTALA (Emergency Medical Treatment and Labor Act) is federal legislation, passed in 1985, requiring hospital emergency departments (EDs) to screen patients who present to the ED and, where necessary, to provide treatment to stabilize patients prior to transferring them to another health facility or to discharging them.[8] The legislation offers no guarantee of payment to physicians or hospitals. If a patient has no insurance, or the patient's insurance refuses to pay for the services, it is unlikely that the hospital and physician will be reimbursed. Individual patients may be billed, but there is substantial evidence that such care often is unpaid (Kane, 2003). The legislation was passed to prevent "patient dumping," a practice by which hospitals refused treatment to patients who could not pay for emergency services. EMTALA is one example of how the United States system imposes or attempts to impose equality – all persons, regardless of their ability to pay, must receive treatment in an emergency condition if they present to any emergency department. Studies have found that EMTALA-related treatment is responsible for a significant portion of bad debt incurred by physicians. Bad debt refers to treatment provided with the expectation that they physician and hospital will be paid but that goes unpaid (Kane, 2003; Young et al., 2002). Bad debt can affect the ability of physicians and hospitals to continue to provide care.

A second way in which the United States attempts to create equality in its health care system is by mandating that health insurance cover specific procedures or treatments. Individual states, which regulate insurance, can require that all health plans offered in the state provide coverage for specific treatments or services. For example, Hawaii and a number of other states require coverage for numerous interventions to address infertility. Other states require coverage of contraceptives, or osteoporosis screenings, or wigs for patients experiencing medically-related hair loss. This means that any insurance plan offered in the state must cover these services; no one may buy insurance coverage that does not include these services in states requiring them. Sometimes mandates are in the form of parity laws. A state may require that insurers that offer coverage for physical conditions must offer comparable coverage for mental health care. The number of mandates has been rising steadily. These mandates raise the cost of insurance, and some studies have suggested that a significant proportion of persons in the United States who lack health insurance would have coverage if such mandates were not in place (Jensen & Morrisey, 1999; Goodman & Musgrave, 1988).[9] If these studies are correct, then part of the uninsured population in the United States could be helped by the abandonment of such mandates.[10] Without mandates, insurance coverage could be less expensive because some plans would not cover some of the procedures or products currently required by mandates. This could mean that more employers would offer some kind of health insurance and that more individuals would opt to pay for health insurance.

Reason 4: Diversity and inequality help avoid the moral hazard of overuse faced by health systems that treat all equally and attempt to provide uniform coverage to all. Any health system, whether public or private, in which persons pay a flat fee for all the care they use gives individuals no incentive to use resources carefully and to seek only the care they need. In such a system, entitlements are created and individuals have an incentive to use anything and everything, since they see themselves as having paid for it and, perhaps, as having a right to it. Markets help people become good decision-makers by providing motives to make good choices.[11] As the Chinese health care system is reformed, great care must be exercised in developing both private and public health systems, including any "safety net" established, to avoid this hazard. Any system that provides consumers no incentive to make careful choices is at risk for being unsustainable because of irresponsible decisions. Some have argued that there is a significant number of individuals in the United States who lack health insurance but who could, in all likelihood, afford it if they chose to forego other expenses (Herrick, 2004; see also United States Department of Commerce, 2003). The decision not to pay for insurance is not altogether unreasonable for such persons. They assume that the care they do need either must be provided regardless of payment, because of EMTALA, or can be obtained for less than the cost of buying insurance. They are willing to "gamble" and assume that they will not incur significant costs for which they will be responsible. Any effort to encourage responsible market choices will involve inequality and diversity and will hold people accountable for those choices.

Despite my claims that it is important to allow for diversity in a health system, it is reasonable to set some limits, or side-constraints, on health care organizations in establishing a health care system. It would be impossible for me to discuss these side-constraints in great detail here. However, I will make some preliminary suggestions. First, health care organizations will have to abide by all applicable laws and regulations in society. The question of what those laws and regulations should be is another matter, though I already have suggested that attempts to regulate the health care industry to require equality of care or equal access to care can be problematic. Second, health care organizations must truthfully disclose their commitments. This is essential in the absence of common commitments. Such disclosure can provide individuals with some sense of what they might expect from an organization and what the organization may expect of them. As I discuss diversity and integrity in health care below, the importance of this will become more evident. Third, organizations generally should respect their oral and written agreements. Again, without this side-constraint, relationships and expectations are unstable.

4 The Importance of Health Care Organizations Maintaining Their Integrity

Once we recognize the importance allowing diverse types of health care organizations to exist, we will recognize that it is important that these institutions maintain their integrity. I defend this claim by explaining what it is for organizations to maintain their integrity. Then I will identify some reasons for which organizational integrity is important.

4.1 Integrity

Although there are several ways one may understand integrity, integrity here refers to coherence between three different aspects of an agent's moral character.[12] (1) First is the stated moral character of an agent, which refers to what that person or organization says it is committed to doing. For example, a person may say he is committed to animal rights, or an organization may say it is committed to caring for the poor. (2) Second is the manifest moral character, which refers to what an agent's actions, decisions, and behaviors suggest are its commitments. For example, an individual might say she is committed to protecting animals from any suffering and to not killing animals for any reason. However, if she wears leather, owns a car with leather seats, and takes medications that have been tested on animals, her actions suggest that her commitment to animals is more limited than she says. Her actions, unlike her value claims or her stated moral character, suggest that she is not deeply opposed to the killing of animals. (3) Third is the deep moral character of an agent, which refers to the agent's fundamental commitments. These commitments define the agent and ought to drive the agent's activities. For example, an individual might be committed to protecting the environment. For an organization, the fundamental commitment might be to religious principles or to innovation and progress or to some other ideal. This sometimes is referred to as an organization's "mission."

Moral integrity measures the coherence among these three aspects of moral character. Integrity refers to an *ordered* coherence, one in which the agent's fundamental moral commitments (deep moral character or mission) are reflected in the agent's value claims (stated moral character) and actions (manifest moral character). In other words, an individual with full moral character integrity is one whose actions and value claims reflect its fundamental commitments.[13]

A few observations about the implications of this understanding of integrity are in order. First, only those individuals or organizations that *have* moral commitments can have moral integrity. If an organization or a person has no particular commitments – no deep moral character – there is nothing against which we may measure its actions and claims. Second, with this understanding of integrity, integrity is a matter of degree – agents may possess more or less integrity as there is more or less overlap between the different aspects of an agent's moral character. Integrity is not a binary condition that an agent either possesses entirely or fails to possess altogether. Third, this understanding of integrity also means that we may make different types of moral judgments about an agent's acts. From the perspective of an agent's moral character we may judge her actions to be wrong. But they may be acceptable from the perspective of general moral norms. For example, in our society there is no general moral norm that says one must donate at least 20% of one's income to the poor. But if one is a member of a religion that requires this, the individual is obligated to fulfill this duty in order to have integrity. We might say that a member of such a religion lacks integrity and acts wrongly if he fails to give his 20%, but we also may say he has not acted immorally from the perspective of social morality. Fourth, and related to the third, insofar as agents have different moral commitments, they will have to live up to different standards to have integrity. For example, a health care organization that includes among its basic commitments a desire always to provide the most advanced, cutting-edge treatments to its patients and an organization committed to meeting the health needs of the poor will have to act very differently to be judged as having integrity. We may say both have integrity even though they provide health care very differently.

Regardless of the nature of an organization's fundamental moral commitments, organizations with full moral integrity might be expected to have the following features. First, they will have some set of fundamental commitments that give them purpose or direction. Second, they will have clear statements concerning their commitments. This is important both for those associated with it and for those contemplating building a relationship with the organization. Where there is diversity, individuals need accurate disclosure so that they can have some sense of what to expect from an organization. Third, individuals who develop the organization's policies must understand the organization's moral character and be committed to ensuring the integrity of the institution. Fourth, individuals who implement, follow and enforce the organization's policies (which should reflect and promote its commitments), namely its executives, professional staff, and other employees, should have an appropriate understanding of the organization's moral commitments, particularly as these relate to their own activities. Such persons should be committed to upholding the institution's deep moral commitments, whether or not they themselves share those commitments. Fifth, the organization will be prepared to evaluate the extent to which its integrity is maintained. The organization must evaluate itself or invite others to do so to determine whether it is acting with integrity. Greater attention is given to specific practices that help foster and maintain integrity below.

4.2 The Importance of Integrity

Thus far I have offered a background for understanding (1) why it is reasonable and prudent to encourage diversity in a health care system and (2) what integrity is. I now discuss the importance of health care organizations maintaining their integrity in a diverse health care system. If through law, regulation, and other forms of social and political pressure, or if through internal dysfunction, an organization fails to maintain its integrity, it may cease to exist altogether – it may not survive because employees may refuse to work for it or patients may refuse to receive health care there or because they organization cannot survive financially. Alternatively, the organization may continue to exist physically, but, without integrity it may not continue to be the same organization in a morally meaningful way. The advantages offered by the existence of diverse types of health care organizations will be lost if they fail to maintain their integrity. In addition to the four advantages of a diverse health care system already noted, consider the following reasons for promoting diversity and integrity in a health care system.

First, in societies that lack universal agreement concerning morality, integrity allows us to make strong normative claims regarding an institution's obligations. We would be unable to make such strong claims without the concepts of moral character and integrity. Particular agents may see themselves as having particular moral obligations that are normative for them even though we may not be justified in asserting that these obligations apply to all agents. Moral obligations of this sort are not universal. Integrity allows us to evaluate the extent to which agents fulfill their obligations even when those obligations are not shared by all. Thus, integrity gives us a richer understanding of moral obligation and allows us to attribute more robust obligations to particular agents than we would be able to attribute in societies lacking universal agreement on the content of morality. Integrity draws on rich cultural and religious traditions to generate particular, content-full moral obligations.

Second, no individual or organization can commit itself to pursing all that is good and valuable. All agents, even those with the best intentions, must choose which goods to pursue and how to pursue them. The world is finite and resources are limited, thus to adopt a particular set of moral aims is to recognize the reality of limitations. For example, it is impossible to provide free health care for the poor who cannot pay and inexpensive care to those who can only afford or choose to pay only for basic care while at the same time providing the most advanced care to all patients. A society benefits from having organizations committed to providing basic care to the poor for free, organizations committed to offering inexpensive basic health care, and organizations committed to advancing medicine.

Third, once agents choose commitments, it is reasonable to want to evaluate the extent to which they fulfill them. This is a sign of taking moral responsibility seriously; we are not merely interested in agents having commitments, we are concerned with the fulfillment of those commitments. Integrity allows us to *judge* the extent to which agents satisfy their obligations.

Fourth, integrity measures internal coherence. We value coherence in itself, as evidence by our general disdain for hypocrisy. We also value coherence because it is related to being fulfilled. Baruch Brody explains the importance of integrity, which he describes as coherence between one's values and one's actions: integrity is "[a] reflection of the way people *should* relate to their values" (1988, p. 90; italics added). Moreover, "We see the formulation of values and goals as a valuable activity but one which would be undercut by a lack of integrity, and we therefore see integrity as something objectively good" (p. 90). Integrity "calls upon health care providers and health care recipients to stand firm in their values. It evaluates choices at least in part on the extent to which those choices are consonant with the personal values of both the provider and the recipient of health care" (p. 37).[14]

Fifth, integrity is a necessary condition for trust in health care, and it often has been argued that it is important for patients to be able to trust physicians, nurses, and health care organizations (Clarke, 2002; Sokowlowski, 1991; Illich, 1975). Trust is the reliable expectation that the one trusted (the trustee) will act in a way that the person trusting (the truster) approves.[15] Thus trust involves both having a reliable basis for projecting how another agent will act and approving of that expected action.[16] Organizational diversity and organizational integrity both are necessary conditions for the possibility of trust in health care.

For there to be any possibility of trust, there must (1) be diverse health care organizations and professionals who hold different commitments and (2) these professionals and organizations must maintain their integrity, that is, they must articulate and act on their fundamental commitments. If there is no diversity among health care organizations, then some individuals will be unable to obtain health care in organizations they can trust because there will not be organizations of whose anticipated actions they approve.[17] There may be deep disagreement that renders individuals unable to trust certain physicians, nurses, or health care organizations even when they have sufficient information to form reliable expectations about their actions. For example, individuals may disagree about how much latitude their families should be given in making health care decisions on their behalf, should they become incompetent. Some patients may want to be able to document their wishes and ensure those wishes are respected regardless of what the family prefers. Others may want to allow their families to make treatment decisions. These two types of patients may not approve of the same health care organization. Some health care organizations, such as those with a strong commitment to the Western conception of patient autonomy, may hold that patient autonomy is a priority and they may seek to require or at least encourage all patients to document their preferences and make decisions based solely on that. Others may hold that patients should not be burdened by completing an advance directive or making treatment decisions. Diversity among providers is important to make it possible for patients with different commitments to trust their physicians and the health care organizations within which they receive care. Trust also requires that diverse organizations maintain their integrity; they must articulate and live out their commitments.[18] Without such integrity, it is impossible for patients to form reliable expectations. For example, if an organization says it is deeply committed to respecting patient autonomy by honoring advanced directives as long as the requests are legal but the organization sometimes acquiesces to family members' demands that violate a patient's advance directive, then patients will not be able to form a reliable expectation about how the organization will act.

In short, to trust a health care organization, patients must be able to expect reliably that the organization will function in some particular way and then they must approve of those anticipated practices. This requires that organizations (1) truthfully disclose their commitments; (2) act on their commitments; and (3) that a diversity of organizations exist so that patients with different priorities and moralities can find organizations of whose commitments and anticipated practices they approve. To be sure, moral integrity is not an absolute moral good. Individuals or organizations may hold morally bad commitments. By articulating those commitments and acting on them, the organization has integrity. But we would not necessarily believe that the organization or individual with integrity was morally good. Nevertheless, there is reason for Chinese policy-makers to be concerned with organizational integrity among Chinese health care organizations because such integrity is important.

5 Maintaining Organizational Integrity

To the extent that they understand organizational diversity and integrity as important elements of an efficient and progressive health care system that promotes responsibility in health care decision-making, that is sustainable, and that makes trust between patients, physicians, and health care organizations possible, Chinese policy makers should be concerned with the preservation of such diversity and integrity. The integrity of diverse organizations can be challenged both from within health care organizations and by society. I turn my attention to considering the ways in which health care organizations can establish their integrity and protect it from external and internal challenges.

5.1 Establish Commitments and Determine their Implications for Organizational Life

First, to have integrity organizations must establish commitments and determine what those commitments mean for the organization. An organization that has no particular commitments or no clear understanding of its commitments cannot have integrity. Sometimes organizations make ambiguous commitments, such as "to respect the dignity of the poor" or "to promote social justice." Much is left to the imagination to determine what it means to respect the dignity of the poor or promote social justice, and different individuals working on behalf of an organization may understand the commitments differently. The implications of these commitments for how the organization should operate must be specified for organizations to maintain their integrity.

In choosing its fundamental commitments, a number of important categories of concern emerge.[19] This list is not exhaustive. It merely illustrates some of the decisions organizations may face in establishing themselves. Notice the importance of culture, tradition, and religion in establishing these commitments.

(1) Will the organization be a secular or belief-based organization? If it will be belief-based, which commitments will be relevant and how will they shape the organization? Compare a religious organization that a loose affiliation to a particular religious with one that has a stronger affiliation. A number of hospitals in the United States have what many would consider loose affiliations to religious groups. These are institutions that have religious roots and often the name of the hospital still appears religious, but the organization itself does not act in a way that marks it as religious or as representing a particular religion. On the other hand are organizations that attempt to maintain a robustly belief-centered environment. Loma Linda University Medical Center (LLUMC), a Seventh-Day Adventist university medical center in southern California, has attempted to keep close ties to its religious identity. LLUMC operates under the guidance of the Seventh-Day Adventist Church's (1988) "Operating Principles for Health-Care Institutions." Some, though not all, of the principles reflect the Seventh-Day Adventist tradition and distinguish the organization from most other health care organizations. For example, Seventh-Day Adventist institutions are to maintain "the sacredness of the Sabbath by promoting a Sabbath atmosphere for staff and patients, avoiding routine business, elective diagnostic services, and elective therapies on Sabbath" (LLUMC, 1988, p. 1). Such institutions should promote "an ovo-lactovegetarian diet free of stimulants and alcohol and an environment free of tobacco smoke" (p. 1, second principle). LLUMC accomplishes this in part by not serving meat or meat products, beverages with caffeine, or alcohol in its cafeterias to promote adherence to Seventh-Day Adventist dietary restrictions (Carr, 2001).[20]

(2) What type of patients will the organization care for? For example, will the organization have a special commitment to the poor, or will it provide concierge care, or care for patients with routine insurance coverage? Will the organization care for patients with very specific conditions, such as a cancer hospital, or will it be a community hospital?

(3) What will be the role of profit in the organization's value and decision-making structure?[21] For example, will the organization seek to ensure a certain level of profitability? If so, how will it do so?

(4) Will the organization serve as a teaching institution? If so, how much priority will be given to providing education versus to providing the best patient care or respecting patients' wishes or interests? Consider the debate over the permissibility of

allowing or even requiring medical students to perform pelvic exams, without consent, on anesthetized women about to undergo gynecologic surgery. At one time this was standard practice in many U.S. medical schools (Annas, 1980; Bewley, 1992; Bibby, Boyd, Redman, & Luesley, 1988; Coney, 1988; Cohen et al., 1989). Some schools changed their practices during the 1990s and required that students obtain consent from patients prior to those patients being anesthetized. Other schools have continued the practice, however, and some have argued that these exams have important educational value and should be permitted without consent (McCullough & Surendran, 2003).[22] If an organization adopts a fundamental commitment to medical education, it may very well hold that fulfilling its teaching mission is more important than obtaining consent for such exams. Organizations that will serve as teaching institutions must determine the extent to which teaching priorities are more important than other values.

(5) Will the organization engage in biomedical research? If so, what priority will be given to research? What types of research will be conducted? Will patients be encouraged to participate in research? Will clinicians in the organization be permitted to enroll their own patients in studies and, if so, under what circumstances? In the United States, most health care organizations that conduct research must ensure that their investigators meet the minimum requirements set forth in the *Code of Federal Regulations.* However, individual organizations may adopt additional requirements or restrictions. Deciding whether any research should be conducted and, if so, any additional limitations the organization might place on research activities are important decisions.

These are only examples of the concerns organizations might consider. In so far as we can imagine more than one reasonable response to the questions raised here, this list demonstrates that a society may have a wide range of health care institutions. Organizations must ensure that their fundamental commitments are sufficiently developed so that they can guide organizational decisions and actions. If an organization's commitments are vague or silent on important matters, they will not be action-guiding for the organization. They also will not help individuals generate reliable expectations about what the organization might do or how it might act.

In establishing commitments, organizations must ensure that their commitments are reasonable. An organization that adopts commitments it knows cannot fulfill or that it will not be called on to fulfill has not established a commitment that is part of its deep moral character. Such an organization is, borrowing Charles Taylor's language, "shallowly sincere" (Taylor, 1991).[23] Part of ensuring that an organization's commitments are reasonable requires consideration of the reality of resource limitations. Organizations should avoid making commitments that cannot be fulfilled because of the finiteness of resources. This is not to suggest that organizations may never adopt a commitment that will be difficult to fulfill and that sometimes may not be fulfilled. Nor is it to restrict organizations to adopting only commitments that they can virtually guarantee they will fulfill without fail. Requiring that would leave us with very thin organizations. In developing their fundamental commitments, organizations must balance the visionary and promissory characteristics of commitments.

Commitments are, to some extent goals that draw an organization forward. They are not meant to stifle an organization, nor are they intended to be so shallow that an organization can fulfill them with little or no effort. At the same time, commitments give others grounds for expecting organizations to act in particular ways; they are, in this sense, public promises. They should not be adopted if it is very unlikely that they can be fulfilled.

Another aspect of ensuring that an organization's commitments are reasonable and can guide organizational behavior in a coherent fashion is ensuring that the organization's commitments are not inherently incompatible. For example, some organizations may say their three primary commitments are to providing high quality patient care, to preparing future physicians and nurses by participating in medical education, and to advancing medicine through research. These commitments may be compatible in many cases. Patients may benefit from being in an organization in which professionals participate in the latest research and in which a cadre of medical students and residents frequently evaluate their health status. In some cases, however, the research and teaching commitments of the organization may diminish the quality of patient care. Thus it may not be possible for an organization to fulfill all of its commitments fully and simultaneously. Such organizations must determine in advance which commitments trump others.

Finally, organizations must determine which commitments are central to an organization's identity and hence integrity. As organizations face challenges to their integrity, they will have to determine which elements of their fundamental commitments are in fact fundamental and essential for maintaining their integrity. In the United States, many health care organizations have religious roots but no longer have explicitly religious commitments. As organizations shed their religious identities, one can question whether they have denigrated their integrity. In some cases, organizations have argued that their religious commitments were not in fact fundamental commitments central to their identity. As a result, they could, they claimed, diminish or altogether abandon their religious identities without violating their integrity. Long Island Jewish Medical Center (LIJMC) is such an organization. It was founded as a Jewish hospital but, despite its name, no longer has a truly Jewish identity. For example, the hospital's synagogue now serves as an inter-faith chapel/meditation room that can accommodate any religious practice or service, including the daily Muslim prayers (Yedvab, 2001). The organization initially cared for the poor immigrant Jewish community in New York. As the Jewish population left the area and no longer needed charity care, other immigrants appeared needing health care. Those immigrants were, by and large, not Jewish. Hence the organization set aside its Jewish identity to fulfill its more basic commitment of serving poor immigrants. The organization maintains that its fundamental commitment to serving the poor of the area actually required that it shed its Jewish identity. Thus it sees itself as having diminished its Jewish identity so that it could fulfill its more basic commitment – so that it could maintain its integrity (Yedvab, 2001).

Whether or not any particular organization is correct in claiming that it may or even must set aside what some may see as a fundamental commitment is a matter of judgment. In some cases, organizations that make such a claim may be wrong; they may violate their integrity by shedding some of their commitments, despite their intentions to maintain their integrity.

5.2 Recognize the Organization's Fundamental Commitments as Normative for the Organization

To establish and maintain their integrity, organizations must ensure that they treat their fundamental commitments as normative. This involves establishing and maintaining an organizational culture that promotes use of an organization's commitments as action-guiding as well as adopting decision processes that intentionally place emphasis on an organization's obligations and duties as grounded in the organization's fundamental commitments. The importance of organizational culture cannot be under-estimated. Janie M. Harden Fritz, Ronald C. Arnett, and Michele Conkel (1999) studied organizational practices to identify the factors that had the greatest impact on determining the extent to which employees acted in accordance with institutions' ethical norms. They found that clearly articulating its commitments and maintaining an environment in which those commitments are respected are central to maintaining organizational integrity. Establishing and maintaining an organizational culture that promotes integrity also requires introducing new employees to an organization's identity and commitments and helping them to understand the implications of those commitments for their work. Even before new employees are hired, they must understand the commitments to determine whether they are compatible with the organization.

In recent years, a number of organizations in the United States have turned to the concept of values-based decision making (VBDM) to promote faithfulness to organizational commitments. VBDM allows organizations to use their basic commitments to guide their decisions and actions. It gives a formal framework for using a set of core values as the primary source of direction and guidance. VBDM calls on organizations and individuals acting on behalf of organizations to treat a mission as action-guiding in a morally binding way. As a result, an organizations claims and actions should reflect its basic commitments – an organization should have integrity.

5.3 Establish Procedures for Navigating Conflict Among Commitments

To maintain their integrity, organizations also must develop procedures for navigating conflicts among their commitments should such conflicts arise. Sometimes resource limitations will make it impossible for an organization to fulfill all of its commitments. For example, imagine an organization that is committed to providing high quality, cutting edge health care to patients. As health care becomes more and more technologically advanced (and expensive), it may not be possible for the organization to offer the most advanced care in all areas. The organization may have to choose between decreasing the range of services offered, finding ways to charge patients more, or providing less-than-the-latest treatments in some areas.

5.4 Respond to Internal and External Challenges to Integrity

Direct threats to an organization's integrity may arise both internally and externally. From within, an organization's integrity may be threatened by individuals associated with the organization, such as leaders, employees, or patients. For example, imagine an organization committed to respecting patient autonomy; honoring patients wishes (as long as those wishes are legal); and communicating clearly with patients about treatment options, recommendations and decisions. A patient insists that should anything happen to him, he wants everything done to resuscitate him, even if it ends up hurting him. The physician thinks the patient should be allowed to die if he experiences a cardiopulmonary arrest because the patient is terminally ill, is in a very weakened state, and the physician believes that any aggressive effort to perform cardiopulmonary resuscitation will be both ineffective and cause the patient physical harm. The physician believes that aggressive attempts to resuscitate this patient are medically inappropriate. The physician explains this to the patient, and the patient insists that he is not ready to die and wants everything done. He asks the physician to promise that he will do everything. The physician informally tells the unit staff that should the patient code, a "slow code" should be done. Slow codes are altered attempts at resuscitation in which health care professionals typically "go through the motions" of a code but do not truly attempt to resuscitate the patient.[24] The physician has failed to uphold the organization's commitment to clear and honest communication with patients and to honoring patients' wishes.

From outside, an organization's integrity may be threatened by social, legal, or financial pressures. I offered earlier the example of state regulation of health insurance companies. States may require that all health insurance sold in the state provide certain kinds of coverage. In some states, for example, one cannot buy health insurance that does not pay for wigs for patients with medically-related hair loss. The result of this is three-fold. First, it raises the cost of health insurance, making it impossible to find a very basic and inexpensive policy. Second, it means that if one finds some particular health service immoral, and the state requires that it be covered, one cannot buy a health insurance policy one finds morally acceptable. Individuals must choose between (a) more expansive coverage that includes services they believe are immoral and thus never will use and (b) no coverage. Or, if one simply does not want to purchase insurance coverage for a procedure or product one has no interest in using, one must choose between paying for coverage that includes it and no coverage at all. Imagine a man who has been bald for the last 27 years. He may very well reason that he has no desire for a wig should he undergo chemotherapy. Yet in many states he may only buy health insurance that would cover the costs of a wig in such circumstances. Imagine telling all car owners that they must purchase insurance coverage that will pay for replacing the convertible top on a vehicle even if they do not own a convertible. Third, it means that an organization committed either to not providing certain forms of health care or to providing very basic, affordable care cannot do so and thus cannot maintain its integrity.

To understand how law and regulation can threaten organizational integrity, consider the 1986 case of Beverly Requena. Requena had amyotrophic lateral sclerosis (ALS) and had been hospitalized repeatedly in St. Clare's/Riverside Medical Center. The organization was a Roman Catholic hospital. Requena's disease had reached a stage at which she would be able to receive nutrition and hydration only artificially; she no longer could swallow. She asked that artificial nutrition and hydration be withheld even though she knew she would die of starvation and dehydration. St. Clare's/Riverside Medical Center claimed that its moral commitments and religious heritage would not permit it to withhold nutrition and hydration from such a patient. Another hospital in the area was willing to accept Requena as patient and was willing to withhold nutrition and hydration, she could be transported safely, and her treating physician would be able to continue to care for her. However, she refused to be transferred, stating that she was otherwise pleased with her care at St. Clare's/Riverside and that she wanted to die there. The court determined that the Catholic hospital had an obligation to withhold nutrition and hydration, in part because forcing Requena to choose between leaving the institution and receiving nutrition and hydration would be "coercive" (*In the matter of Beverly Requena*, Superior Court of New Jersey – Chancery Division, Morris County, P-326-86E, September 24, 1986; *In the Matter of Beverly Requena*, Superior Court of New Jersey – Appellate Division, A-442-86T5, October 6, 1986). The organization clearly held that to withhold nutrition and hydration in this case violated its fundamental moral commitments – its integrity – but it was obligated to do so anyway by the state.[25]

Thus far I have focused on the benefits of having diverse health care organizations in a society, the importance of such organizations maintaining their integrity, and I have considered some of the ways in which organizations can maintain their integrity. I turn my attention now to some of the concerns and conflicts that arise when diverse health care organizations exist within a society.

6 Concerns that Arise when Organizations have Different Models and Standards of Ideal Behavior

6.1 The Interests and Priorities of the State and Certain Private Organizations may Conflict

Private health care organizations may have commitments different from those of the state. This in itself is not problematic, but sometimes their commitments may come into direct conflict with the interests of the state. For example, in the United

States pharmaceutical products and medical devices must be approved by the Food and Drug Administration (FDA) before they can be sold in the United States.[26] There are products that have not yet been reviewed and approved by the FDA or that have been reviewed and disapproved by the FDA and thus are unavailable in the US. Sometimes they may be available in other countries. Even if some believe the products are promising or are willing to take the risk, the FDA prohibits health care professionals and organizations from making such drugs or devices available to patients (outside the context of clinical trials) in the United States for two main reasons. The state is committed to (1) protecting the public overall from drugs and devices whose risks the government deems are greater than their benefits and (2) gathering sufficient data from controlled clinical trials so that it can review drugs and devices for potential approval. If unapproved drugs or devices were available outside clinical trials, it might take much longer to gather data. I will say more about this later.

One can imagine a health care organization committed to serving patients with a disorder for which there is no known effective treatment or for which the known effective treatments have terrible side-effects and risks. Such patients may believe that it is rational to use new drugs that have not yet been approved or drugs disapproved by the FDA but that are in use elsewhere. They are willing to assume risks for the possibility of benefit. Much has been written about the personal nature of risk-benefit judgments; the levels of risk individuals are willing to assume for a potential benefit is a personal decision. Assessing risks and benefits is a subjective activity; it blends science and judgment with psychological, social, cultural, and political factors (Slovic, 1999, p. 689). We have seen how desperately ill patients often are willing to assume the risk of taking a drug whose benefits are not yet known and whose risks may be great because they have no other option and without the drug they certainly will die. This was the case in the 1980s as AIDS treatments were being developed. HIV/AIDS advocates wanted research to move quickly but they also want to ensure access to medications under development. Patients were willing to take drugs whose benefits were not known and whose risks and side-effects might be tremendous because the alternative death sentence seemed worse.[27] The desire of such to use a product that is not approved, whose benefits or risks are unknown, or whose risks/side-effects appear to many to outweigh the potential benefits are not necessarily irrational or ignorant. Unlike other people, they know they are dying and that a painful death almost certainly awaits them. Thus they are willing to take a chance on a new product. If it fails to help them, they probably will not be worse off than they already are. And if it happens to provide any benefit, they will be better off. The potential side effects and risks do not outweigh the potential benefits *for them*.

Individual health care organizations serving such patients may seek to grant them access to unapproved drugs or devices. One can imagine an organization that holds a fundamental commitment to patients in danger of dying soon and to serving their interests and allowing them to make health care decisions etc.[28] Allowing access to unapproved medications and devices conflicts with the interest of the state. Thus a health care organization that wants to serve such patients has a commitment that conflicts with the interest of the state. It is in the interest of the state (and of society overall) that patients be allowed open access (outside a trial) only to drugs and devices that have been tested and approved and it is in the interest of the state (and society) that new products be tested in the context of controlled trials to ensure that there is sufficient data to approve or disapprove a new product. If open access is granted outside the context of trials, then there may be insufficient data to determine whether or not a treatment is effective.

This is precisely what happened when physicians thought patients with advanced breast cancer might benefit from high-dose chemotherapy followed by bone marrow transplants. During the mid-1980s and into the late 1990s, many women with advance breast cancer were treated outside the context of a clinical trial with high-dose chemo-therapy followed by bone marrow transplantation. Although clinical trials for this intervention were open, many women sought treatment outside the trial context to avoid randomization, i.e., to ensure that they received the "new treatment." Through the courts, many insurance carriers were forced to pay for the unproven intervention. It eventually was show that the "treatment" was ineffective (Dresser, 2001, pp. 61–62). This determination could have been made years earlier had the "treatment" been offered only in the context of controlled clinical trials. There were tremendous costs to society and the state associated with providing the intervention outside the context of trials. But the patients themselves were not necessarily irrational for wanting access to the intervention. For them – women who had a disease that had progressed to the point that they were unlikely to survive – it might very well have been worth the risk. (It was not necessarily worth the risk of paying for ineffective treatment to society. There is a difference between saying that an individual is not being unreasonable for wanting to use an intervention that is unproven and saying that society should be willing to pay for it. In making choices about what treatments to cover, private and public payers of health care make judgments about what treatments are more likely than others to provide benefit. Thus there is nothing irrational about saying that society is not willing to bear the cost burden of an unproven, unapproved treatment while at the same time saying that it is rational for a patient to want the intervention.)[29]

Being permitted legal access to an intervention through a private health care organization when such access conflicts with the interest of the state is what is of interest here. Determining how to address such conflicts is a matter of public policy. Given the advantages of having diverse organizations that maintain their integrity, there should be an interest in minimizing infringement on their integrity. However, as I said earlier, integrity is not an absolute value. Insofar as infringement on organizational integrity is essential for security, regulating services or providing services directly through government organizations may be appropriate. Beyond that, however, one should recognize the advantages individuals, organizations, and society overall experience when health care organizations with different commitments exist. It also is in the interests of individuals, society, and organizations that organizations disclose their commitments and maintain their integrity. Failure to do so may make it harder to maintain their integrity both because individuals affiliated with organizations may not know what is required of them and they may act in ways that violate their integrity. Moreover, individuals who do not know about an organization's commitments and affiliate with it may learn that they disapprove of the organization's commitments and intentionally act against those commitments.

6.2 The Lack of Uniform Standards may Make it Difficult for Patients and Health Care Professionals to Understand the Commitments of Particular Health Care Organizations

In a society in which different health care organizations have different commitments and treat similar cases differently, there is concern that patients' or employees' expectations may be distorted and may make decisions that are contrary to their own interests because of such misunderstandings. The 1986 case of Beverly Requena discussed earlier serves as an example. The Court held that the patient, at the time of admission, did not understand the implications of being hospitalized in that facility (*In the matter of Beverly Requena*, Superior Court of New Jersey – Chancery Division, Morris County, P-326-86E, September 24, 1986; *In the Matter of Beverly Requena*, Superior Court of New Jersey – Appellate Division, A-442-86T5, October 6, 1986). If all hospitals were committed either to withholding nutrition and hydration in such cases or to providing interventions in such cases, the patient most likely would have known what to expect and the battle that ensued over her decision would have been avoided.

Consider another example. A physician may affiliate with a hospital without realizing the extent to which cost will be a factor in treatment decisions. If the organization is a for-profit institution committed to avoiding any uncompensated care, the physician may be prohibited from offering procedures for which payment is not guaranteed. If the physician believes that money should not be an overriding factor in medical decision making, the physician may find working in that organization morally compromising.

In a society in which all health care organizations have comparable fundamental commitments, i.e., in which there was no significant diversity among health care organizations, such confusion would not arise. However, to require uniformity among organizations is to lose the advantages associated with diversity and competition.

It is, no doubt, important for patients, prospective patients, employees, and prospective employees to understand the nature of an organization's commitments and their implications. The solution, however, is not to require uniformity. It is to allow organizations to maintain their integrity and require that they disclose truthfully their commitments. Individuals will come to understand that not all organizations are created equally and that they are responsible for making informed decisions when affiliating with health care organizations as patients or employees.

6.3 There may be People Within a Society Who Object to the Existence of Certain Kinds of Health Care Organizations

In a society in which individuals have different conceptions of morality or merely different health care priorities, there may be individuals who object to the existence of certain kinds of health care organizations. Consider the example of MergerWatch. MergerWatch "monitors the threats to reproductive health care from mergers and other health care industry transactions through which restrictive religious rules are imposed on previously secular health care providers and services are banned" (MergerWatch, 2002). Much of their attention has been on mergers between Catholic and non-Catholic health care organizations in the United States because Catholic facilities generally participate in mergers only if the newly formed organization will have a Catholic identity. MergerWatch has attempted to use legislative support to prevent such mergers and to obligate Catholic hospitals to provide services Catholic hospitals would not voluntarily provide, such as abortions and sterilizations (Kerry, 1999). MergerWatch and the American Civil Liberties Union (ACLU) have encouraged lawmakers to require that Catholic hospitals provide abortions or not receive any federal funding.[30] These groups actively work to limit diversity because they find health care organizations with certain commitments objectionable. Consider another example: In the United States, the practice of retainer medicine or boutique care, allows patients to pay for better access to their physicians, more time with a physician, avoid waiting for an appointment etc. Some members of our society have argued that such practices are unfair and unjust and ought to be prohibited. They hold that individuals who seek such advantages and are willing to pay for them should not be granted such services and organizations seeking to serve such patients should be prohibited from doing so. Such persons find boutique or retainer medicine objectionable and seek to eliminate such organizations from the health care system (Carroll, 2003).

Insofar as health care organizations adhere to the minimal side-constraints imposed by a society, the dissatisfaction of some will not be grounds for justifying the coercion of others or the violation of an organization's commitments and hence integrity. To obtain the advantages associated with a society in which there are different types of health care organizations, diversity will have to flourish. Some personal dissatisfaction with such diversity will be inevitable. Such dissatisfaction would not be eliminated by requiring uniformity. Even in such a system, some would be dissatisfied with the uniform policy adopted.

7 Conclusion

Societies in which diverse types of health care organizations with different and sometimes competing commitments are likely to see (1) technological progress and advancement in health care, (2) a government system that is less burdened, (3) individuals who are careful health care consumers, and (4) individuals who can trust health care organizations. Thus, as China reforms its health care system, it is reasonable and prudent to encourage a diverse health system. To experience the benefits of such diversity, the organizations that compose the health care system must maintain their integrity. That is, they must establish their fundamental commitments, articulate them truthfully, and allow those commitments to guide their actions. Markets facilitate this diversity and integrity; for markets permit the existence of different types of health care organizations and hold organizations accountable for fulfilling their commitments. The combination of diversity and integrity in a market system makes it possible for tradition, religion, and culture to thrive. Organizations adopt particular, content-full moral commitments and must abide by and fulfill them in order to maintain their integrity. Failure to maintain integrity is a failure to fulfill a promise, and markets discourage such behavior. At times, it may be difficult for health care organizations to maintain their integrity, but it is important for them to respond both to internal and external challenges in a way that fosters integrity. There may be times at which commitments of particular health care organizations conflict with the interests of the state or with the interests of particular members of society. Societies must make an effort to encourage organizations to maintain their integrity even in such cases, insofar as possible, if the society is to experience the benefits of a diverse health system. A thick conception of integrity such as this is a resource for maintaining traditional cultural and religious commitments and avoiding moral vacuity.

Notes

1 Much of the material discussed here was developed in Iltis (2001a, 2001b, 2003, 2004, 2005a).

2 The American Medical Association (AMA) issued a report on boutique medicine in June, 2002. The report concludes that the AMA "currently finds no evidence that special physician-patient contracts, such as retainer agreements, adversely impact the quality of patients' care or the access of any group of patients to care" (2002, p. 5). The practice is becoming increasingly common in the United States. The American Society of Concierge Physicians (2004), now called The Society for the Innovative Practice of Medicine, estimates that there are hundreds of practices in the United States following different concierge care models.

3 These guidelines are the *Ethical and Religious Directives for Catholic Health Care Services* published by the United States Conference of Catholic Bishops (2001).

4 For a discussion of Loma Linda University, see Covrig (2001, 2003).

5 Estimates vary as to how many Canadians actually obtain health care in the United States (Katz, Cardiff, Pascali, Barer, & Evans, 2002; Korcok, 1991, 1997). Some suggest that very few Canadians obtain health care in the United States (Katz et al., 2002) and others suggest the use is significant and likely to increase (Korcok, 1991, 1997).

6 Computerized medication systems are expensive and, although many believe they do reduce medical errors (e.g., Benjamin, 2003; Kaushal (2003); Kaushal, Shojania, & Bates, 2004; Bates et al., 1999), others are concerned that such systems may create other problems (e.g., Graber, 2004).

7 For a discussion of pharmaceutical and biotechnology development in the United States, Europe and Japan with special attention to the impact of policy on innovation, see Lasagna (1996).

[8] EMTALA legislation states that:

> In the case of a hospital that has an emergency department, if any individual (whether or not eligible for Medicare benefits and regardless of ability to pay) comes by him or herself or with another person to the emergency department and a request is made on the individual's behalf for examination or treatment of a medical condition by qualified medical personnel (as determined by the hospital in its rules and regulations), the hospital must provide for an appropriate medical screening examination within the capability of the hospital's emergency department, including ancillary services routinely available to the emergency department, to determine whether or not an emergency medical condition exists. The examinations must be conducted by individuals determined qualified by hospital bylaws or rules and regulations and who meet the requirements of 482.55 concerning emergency services personnel and direction. (42 CFR 489.24)

[9] For information on insurance mandates in different states, see www.statehealthfacts.org

[10] One should note that the problem of uninsured individuals in the United States often is labeled a "crisis." However, this characterization has been challenged by some. For example, Herrick (2004) points out that 84% of the population in the United States either has private insurance or is enrolled in a government health program. This amounts to approximately 243.3 million people. Another 10–14 million people qualify for government programs but have not enrolled. Another 15 million have household incomes over $50,000 but do not have insurance; many of these individuals most likely choose not to pay for insurance but could afford to do so. Thus it is about 6% of the population that has no insurance, does not qualify for government insurance and earns less than $50,000 per year (Herrick, 2004). These statistics are found in U.S. Department of Commerce (2003).

[11] To be sure, many have been critical of using the market model in health care. For further discussion of health care markets, see Cherry (2003), Menzel (2003), Meadowcroft (2003), Cohen and Burg (2003), Trotter (2003), AMA (1997), Benner (1998), Engelhardt (1991), Engelhardt and Rie (1992).

[12] This understanding of integrity is related to those who have argued that integrity refers to consistency or coherence between an agent's actions and her commitments (Williams, 1973; Brody, 1988), particularly in the face of adversity (Putnam, 1996), or consistency between an agent's actions and her true self (authenticity) (Taylor, 1991, pp. 36–29; Kekes, 1983; Martin, 1991; Van Hooft, 1995; Fuss, 1964).

[13] Sometimes agents may display or possess only partial character integrity. For example, an agent may have a fundamental moral commitment and articulate it clearly. Thus there is coherence between its deep moral character and its stated moral character. But if an agent's actions do not reflect those commitments, then it lacks full integrity.

[14] Despite the importance he grants to integrity, Brody holds that integrity is not an absolute good; it is a value among others that can be overridden (1988, p. 54, n. 62).

[15] I developed and defended this account in a presentation at the American Society for Bioethics and Humanities (Iltis, 2004).

[16] Note that the expectation may not be that the physician, nurse, or health care organization always will act in the trustee's interests. Several accounts of trust in health care call on the trustee to act in the truster's interest (Gambetta, 1998; Jones, 1996; Mechanic, 1998; Illingworth, 2002). These conceptions of trust often will make patients unwarranted in trusting physicians and health care organizations. In reality, physicians and health care organizations often cannot and should not act in a given patient's interest. In part this is because there may be conflict between the interests of a particular physician's or hospital's different patients and in part this is because a given patient's interest may conflict with each other. For example, imagine that Mr. A and Mr. B both have been patients of City Hospital for years. They both were born there, their children have been born there, they have used the emergency department, and had diagnostic testing and surgery there. They have been satisfied with their care. Now imagine that both say they trust the organization, meaning that they both expect that it will act in their interests. Mr. A and Mr. B are driving in the same area and have a car accident. Both are badly injured, need the attention of a trauma surgeon, and need blood

transfusions. It is not possible for them both to be treated simultaneously in the hospital. There is no other hospital nearby and no helicopter available to transport one of the men. Both are taken to City Hospital, but only one is likely to receive sufficient care in time to live. Their interests conflict. It is in each patient's interest to be the one treated. Any definition of trust that depends on expectations about the satisfaction of patients' interests will render trust weak; patients often are unwarranted in expecting that a physician or organization will act in their interest. Sometimes it is wrong for physicians or organizations to act in a particular patient's interest.

There even is disagreement about what constitutes good medical practice and hence what it means to act in a patient's medical interest. Thus we should not be surprised that some trust a particular organization and others distrust it even if all parties have the same information. To understand the disagreement that exits over what constitutes good medical practice, consider the difference between allopathic, homeopathic, osteopathic, and ayurvedic physicians and the extent to which various persons are or are not willing to recognize members of some of those classes as doctors. Note that even physicians who practice within the same school of medicine may disagree. For example, there is tremendous disagreement among allopathic physicians in the United States about whether antibiotics should routinely be prescribed to otherwise-healthy children who have ear infections.

17 If we granted individuals a positive right to have organizations that met their interests exist and be supported, then individuals would be justified in demanding of others that they support such organizations. This could degrade the integrity of other individuals and organizations, since they might be forced to support organizations whose commitments violate their own commitments. In other words, they might be forced violate their own integrity. Thus individuals may claim justifiably only a right of forbearance. Persons do not have a right to force others to be complicit in activities that might violate their own integrity.

18 For further discussion of informed consent, see Fan (1997).

19 This is based on Iltis (2005a).

20 For further discussion of LLUMC and Seventh-Day Adventist institutions in general, see Covrig (2001, 2003). Covrig suggests that LLUMC has attempted to make its founding identity legitimate to a broader range of people and that, in doing so, it has placed its identity at risk (2001).

21 In the United States there is disagreement about whether it is permissible for health care organizations to be explicitly for-profit. Some hold that no health care organization should be specifically for-profit (e.g., Yarborough, 1986; Dougherty, 1990) and others hold that profit is a legitimate motive as long as it is not the organization's primary focus (e.g., Werhane, 2000).

22 In Spring, 2003 debate over this issue broke out in the academic and popular presses. A February, 2003 study in the *American Journal of Obstetrics and Gynecology* (Ubel, Jepson, & Silver-Isenstad, 2003) showed that students' views about the importance of consent changed during the course of their ob/gyn clerkships. Prior to their clerkships medical students typically thought consent should be obtained from patients prior to being anesthetized. After their clerkships far fewer students thought consent was necessary. The authors suggested that students became enculturated to show less respect for patients' right to informed consent. On April 25, 2003, the American College of Obstetrics and Gynecology issued a statement that included the following:

> If a pelvic examination(s) that is planned for an anesthetized woman undergoing surgery offers her no personal benefit and is performed solely for teaching purposes, it should be performed only with her specific informed consent, obtained when she has full decision-making capacity. (ACOG, 2003).

23 For further discussion of the importance of adopting commitments of a particular sort, see Halfon (1989, pp. 16–19).

24 For further discussion, see Tomlinson and Brody (1990), Neher (1988), Gazelle (1998).

25 For further discussion of this case, see Wear (1991).

26 Products that are approved by the FDA for one use may end up be used for other purposes "off label." But they must first be approved for some specific use to be brought to the market.

27 For further discussion, see Dresser (2001) and Epstein (1996).

[28] One should not dismiss too quickly the position of such patients. They are not necessarily blind to the possibility that the drug may not work and may even kill them. If they were enrolled in research, one might think that they are blinded by the therapeutic misconception. The therapeutic misconception refers to patients who are enrolled as subjects in research and mistakenly think that in research the physician will act only with the intention of benefiting them, or that their research participation is a continuation of their clinical care and will be of benefit to them, or that interventions offered through research represented the most up to date and effective treatments and offer them the greatest benefit (Appelbaum, Roth, & Lidz, 1982, 1987). The patients I am describing here do not necessarily think a product will work nor do they necessarily think that being in research will benefit them. They also are not individuals enrolled in a placebo-controlled trial in which they might be receiving a placebo while thinking that they certainly are receiving study medication. Rather they are individuals who have a very different conception of risks and benefits because they are dying. It is not that they have false expectations; for them, the risks associated with a new product are irrelevant compared to the risks of doing nothing.

[29] For a discussion of the role of third party payers in funding biomedical research, see Iltis (2005b).

[30] Federal funding includes Medicaid. Because many Catholic hospitals serve poor populations who receive Medicaid, such organizations would be financially devastated by such a requirement.

References

American College of Obstetricians and Gynecologists (2003). *ACOG Statement: Statement of the ACOG committee on ethics regarding ethical implications of pelvic examination training* [On-line]. Available: http://www.acog.org/from_home/publications/press_releases/nr04-25-03.cfm. Accessed August 9, 2005.

American Medical Association, & Ad Hoc Committee to Defend Health Care. (1997). For our patients, not for profits. *Journal of the American Medical Association, 278*, 1733–1738.

American Medical Association (2002). *Report of the council on medical services.* CMS Report 9-A-02 (June). Available: http://www.ama-assn.org/ama1/pub/upload/mm/372/cms902.rtf. Accessed August 9, 2005.

American Society of Concierge Physicians. (2004). *Patient financed medicine: Past, present and future* [On-line]. Available: http://www.Conciergephysicians.org/GAO%20Report.pdf. Accessed August 9, 2005.

Annas, G. J. (1980). The care of private patients in teaching hospitals. *Bulletin of the New York Academy of Medicine, 56*, 403–411.

Appelbaum, P., Roth, L., & Lidz, C. (1982). The therapeutic misconception: Informed consent in psychiatric research. *International Journal of Law and Psychiatry, 5*, 319–329.

Appelbaum, P., Roth, L., & Lidz, C. (1987). False hopes and best data: Consent to research and the therapeutic misconception. *Hastings Center Report, 17*(2), 20–24.

Bates, D. W., Teich, J. M., Lee, J., Seger, D., Kuperman, G. J., Ma'Luf, N., Boyle, D., & Leape, L. (1999). The impact of computerized physician order entry on medication error prevention. *Journal of American Medical Informatics Association, 6*(4), 313–321.

Benjamin, D. M. (2003). Reducing medication errors and increasing patient safety: Case studies in clinical pharmacology. *Journal of Clinical Pharmacology, 43*, 768–783.

Benner, P. (1998). When health care becomes a commodity: The need for compassionate strangers. In J. Kilner, R. D. Orr, & J. A. Shelly (Eds.), *The changing face of health care* (pp. 119–144). Grand Rapids: Eerdsmans Publishing Company.

Bewley, S. (1992). The law, medical students and assault. *British Medical Journal, 304*, 1551–1553.

Bibby, J., Boyd, N., Redman, C. W., Luesley, D. M. (1988, November 12). Consent for vaginal examination by students on anaesthetized patients. *The Lancet, 2*(8620), 1150.

Brody, B. A. (1988). *Life and death decision making.* New York: Oxford University Press.

Carr, M. (2001, April 2). Personal communication.
Carroll, J. (2003). Concierge care by any other name raises ethical concerns. *Managed Care, 12*(11), 48–51.
Cherry, M. J. (2003). Scientific excellence, professional virtue, and the profit motive: The market and health care reform. *The Journal of Medicine and Philosophy, 28*(3), 259–280.
Clarke, C. C. (2002). Trust in Medicine. *The Journal of Medicine and Philosophy,* 27(1), 11–29.
Cohen, J., & Burg, E. (2003). On the possibility of a positive-sum game in the distribution of health care resources. *The Journal of Medicine and Philosophy, 28*(3), 327–338.
Cohen, D. L., Kessel, R. W., McCullough, L. B., Apostolides, A. Y., Heiderich, K. J., & Alden, E. R. (1989). Pelvic examinations by medical students. *American Journal of Obstetrics and Gynecology, 161*, 1013–1014.
Coney, S. (1988). *The unfortunate experiment*. New York: Penguin Books.
Covrig, D. M. (2001). Stability and change in the religious organizational identify of Loma Linda University. *Research on Christian Higher Education, 8*, 45–68.
Covrig, D. M. (2003). Institutional integrity through periods of significant change. In A. S. Iltis (Ed.), *Institutional integrity in health care* (pp. 139–174). Dordrecht: Kluwer Academic Publishers.
Dougherty, C. J. (1990). The costs of commercial medicine. *Theoretical Medicine, 11*(4), 275–286.
Dresser, R. (2001). *When science offers salvation*. New York: Oxford University Press.
Emergency Medical Treatment and Labor Act (EMTALA) 42 CFR 489.24.
Engelhardt, H. T., Jr. (1991). Virtue for hire: Some reflections on free choice and the profit motive in the delivery of health care. In T. Bole & W. Bondeson (Eds.), *Rights to health care* (pp. 327–353). Dordrecht: Kluwer Academic Publishers.
Engelhardt, H. T. Jr., & Rie, M. (1992). Selling virtue: Ethics as a profit-maximizing strategy in health care delivery. *Journal of Health and Social Policy, 4*, 27–35.
Epstein, S. (1996). *Impure science: AIDS, activism, and the politics of knowledge*. Berkeley: University of California Press.
Fan, R. (1997). Self-determination vs. family-determination: Two incommensurable measures of autonomy. *Bioethics, 11*, 309–322.
Fuss, P. (1964). Conscience. *Ethics,* 74, 111–120.
Gambetta, D. (Ed.). (1998). *Trust: Making and breaking cooperative relations*. New York: Blackwell.
Gazelle, G. (1998). The slow code: Should anyone rush to its defense? *New England Journal of Medicine, 338*(7), 467–469.
Goodman, J. C., & Musgrave, G. L. (1988). Freedom of choice in health insurance. *National Center for Policy Analysis Study No. 134.*
Graber, M. (2004). The safety of computer-based medication systems. *Archives of Internal Medicine, 164*(3), 339–340.
Halfon, M. (1989). *Integrity: A philosophical investigation*. Philadelphia: Temple University Press.
Harden Fritz, J. M., Arnett, R. C., & Conkel, M. (1999). Organizational ethical standards and organizational commitment. *Journal of Business Ethics, 20*, 289–299.
Herrick, D. (2004). *Is there a crisis of the uninsured?* Dallas: National Center for Policy Analysis [On-line]. Available: http://www.ncpa.org/edo/uninsured082604.htm. Accessed August 9, 2005.
Illich, I. (1975). *Medical nemesis: The expropriation of health.* London: Marion Boyers, Ltd.
Illingworth, P. (2002). Trust: The scarcest of medical resources. *The Journal of Medicine and Philosophy,* 27(1), 31–46.
Iltis, A. S. (2001a). Organizational ethics and institutional integrity. *HEC Forum, 13*(4), 317–328.
Iltis, A. S. (2001b). Institutional integrity in Roman Catholic health care institutions. *Christian Bioethics, 7*(1), 93–104.
Iltis, A. S. (2003). A philosophical exploration of the possibility and implications of institutional moral agency. (Doctoral dissertation, Houston: Rice University).

Iltis, A. S. (2004, October 29). *Trust in medicine*. Presentation at the American Society for Bioethics and Humanities, Philadelphia, PA.

Iltis, A. S. (2005a). Values based decision making: Organizational mission and integrity. *HEC Forum, 17*(1), 6–17.

Iltis, A. S. (2005b). Third party payers and the costs of biomedical research. *Kennedy Institute of Ethics Journal, 15*(2), 135–160.

In the Matter of Beverly Requena No.P-326-86E. (1986, September 24). Superior Court of New Jersey, Chancery Division, Morris County.

In the Matter of Beverly Requena No. A-442-86T5. (1986, October 6). Superior Court of New Jersey, Appellate Division.

Jensen, G. A., & Morrisey, M. A. (1999). *Mandated benefit laws and employer-sponsored health insurance*. Washington, DC: Health Insurance Association of American.

Jones, K. (1996). Trust as an affective attitude. *Ethics, 107*, 4–25.

Kane, C. K. (2003). *Physician marketplace report: The impact of EMTALA on physician practices*. Chicago: American Medical Association – Center for Health Policy Research [On-line]. Available: http://www.ama-assn.org/ama1/pub/upload/mm/363/pmr2003-02.pdf. Accessed August 9, 2005.

Katz, S. J., Cardiff, K., Pascali, M., Barer, M. L., & Evans, R. G. (2002). Phantoms in the snow: Canadians' use of health care services in the United States. *Health Affairs, 21*(3), 19–31.

Kaushal, R. (2003). Effects of computerized physician order entry and clinical decision support systems on medication safety: A systematic review. *Archives of Internal Medicine, 163*, 1409–1416.

Kaushal, R., Shojania, K. G., & Bates, D.W. (2004). In reply (to 'The safety of computer-based medication systems' by Mark Graber). *Archives of Internal Medicine, 164*, 340.

Kekes, J. (1983). Constancy and purity. *Mind, 92*, 499–518.

Kerry, J. M. (1999). *MergerWatch: It may be coming to a community near you*. Catholic Health World [On-line]. Available: http://www.chausa.org/PUBS/PUBSART.ASP?ISSUE=W990401&ARTICLE=D. Accessed December 19, 1999.

Korcok, M. (1991). U.S. cash registers humming as Canadian patients flock south. *Canadian Medical Association Journal, 144*(6), 745–747.

Korcok, M. (1997). Excess demand meets excess supply as referral companies link Canadian patients, US hospitals. *Canadian Medical Association Journal, 157*(6), 676–770.

Lasagna, L. (1996). Comparison of U.S., European, and Japanese policies affecting pharmaceutical and biotechnology development. In F. B. Rudolph & L. V. McIntire (Eds.), *Biotechnology: Science, engineering, and ethical challenges for the twenty-first century* (pp. 225–231). Washington, DC: Joseph Henry Press.

Martin, M. W. (1991). Honesty with oneself. In M. Bochover (Ed.), *Rules, rituals, and responsibility* (pp. 115–136). LaSalle, IL: Open Court.

McCullough, M., & Surendran, A. (2003). *Pelvic-exam debate starts with consent: Invasion vs. routine education* [On-line]. Available: http://www.philly.com/mld/inquirer/5357547.htm?template=contentModules/printstory.jsp. Accessed April 23, 2003.

Meadowcroft, J. (2003). The British National Health Service: Lessons from the "socialist calculation debate." *The Journal of Medicine and Philosophy, 28*(3), 307–326.

Mechanic, D. (1998). The functions and limitations of trust in the provision of medical care. *Journal of Health Politics, Policy and Law, 23*, 661–686.

Menzel, P. T. (2003). How compatible are liberty and equality in structuring a health care system. *The Journal of Medicine and Philosophy, 28*(3), 281–306.

MergerWatch (2002). *Home page* [On-line]. Available: http://www.mergerwatch.org. Accessed April 23, 2003.

Neher, J. O. (1988). The "slow code": A hidden conflict. *Journal of Family Practice, 27*(4), 429–430.

Putnam, D. (1996). Integrity and moral development. *Journal of Value Inquiry, 30*(1–2), 237–246.

Seventh-Day Adventist Church. (1988). *Operating principles for health-care institutions* [On-line]. Statement released by the General Conference of Seventh-Day Adventists Executive Committee at the Annual Council session in Nairobi, Kenya in October, 1988. Available: http://www.adventist.org/beliefs/main_stat31.html. Accessed August 9, 2005.

Slovic, P. (1999). Trust, emotion, sex, politics, and science: Surveying the risk-assessment battlefield. *Risk Analysis* 19(4), 689–701.

Sokowlowski, R. (1991). The fiduciary relationship and the nature of the professions. In E. D. Pellegrino, R. Veatch, & J. Langan (Eds.), *Ethics, trust, and the professions* (pp. 23–43). Washington, DC: Georgetown University Press.

Taylor, C. (1991). *The Ethics of authenticity.* Cambridge: Harvard University Press.

Tomlinson, T., & Brody, H. (1990). Futility and the ethics of resuscitation. *Journal of the American Medical Association, 264*(1), 1276–1280.

Trotter, G. (2003). Holding civic medicine accountable: Will Morreim's liability scheme work in a disaster? *The Journal of Medicine and Philosophy, 28*(3), 339–357.

Ubel, P. A., Jepson, C., & Silver-Isenstad, A. (2003). Don't ask, don't tell: A change in medical student attitudes after obstetrics/gynecology clerkships toward seeking consent for pelvic examinations on anesthetized patients. *American Journal of Obstetrics and Gynecology, 188*(2), 575–579.

United States Conference of Catholic Bishops (2001). *The ethical and religious directives for catholic health care services* (4th ed.). [On-line]. Available: http://www.usccb.org/ bishops/directives.shtml. Accessed August 9, 2005.

United States Department of Commerce. (2003). *Income, poverty and health insurance coverage in the United States.* (Authored by Carmen DeNavas-Walt, Bernadette Proctor, & Robert Mills.). Washington: Government Printing Office.

Van Hooft, S. (1995). Integrity and the inchoate self. *Philosophy Today,* 39(3–4), 245–262.

Wear, S. (1991). The moral significance of institutional integrity. *The Journal of Medicine and Philosophy, 16*, 225–230.

Werhane, P. H. (2000). Business ethics, stakeholder theory, and the ethics of healthcare organizations. *Cambridge Quarterly of Healthcare Ethics,* 9, 169–181.

Williams, B. (1973). A critique of utilitarianism. In J. J. C. Smart & B. Williams (Eds.), *Utilitarianism: For and against* (pp. 76–150). London: Cambridge University Press.

Yarborough, M. (1986). Patients and profits. *Theoretical Medicine, 7*, 93–102.

Yedvab, J. (2001, 15 February). Personal Communication.

Young, G. P., Ellis, J., Becher, J., Yeh, C., Kovar, J., & Levitt, M. A. (2002). Managed care gatekeeping, emergency medicine coding, and insurance reimbursement outcomes for 980 emergency department visits from four states nationwide. *Annals of Emergency Medicine, 39*, 24–30.

A Reconstructionist Confucian Approach to Chinese Health Care

The Ethical Principles, the Market, and Policy Reforms

Ruiping Fan

1 The Challenges of Health Care in Current China

The world is witnessing a rapid development of current China – its booming economy, promising markets, advancing sciences and technologies, and improving education, etc. However, China also faces enormous cultural, social and economic problems and difficulties. This paper focuses on issues in Chinese health care ethics, markets, and policies. Let me begin by summarizing a series of severe challenges that China is confronting in the demand and supply of health care as follows.

1. How should China adequately establish and stabilize a sustainable health care system for a huge population with an ever increasing portion of the retired elderly (demanding high-intensity health care interventions) and an ever decreasing portion of the working people (providing funds to support health care)? This is a crucially important issue for the long-term development of Chinese health care system,[1] being all the more urgent with the "four-two-one" structure of the current Chinese family under the government's "one child per couple" population-control policy.
2. What should be done to set up a basic health care delivery accessible to the Chinese peasants in the countryside? Indeed, between the urban and rural areas of current China, there exists an unfair "one country, two systems" in health care delivery: compared to their fellow citizens in cities, Chinese peasants receive much fewer health care funds, investments and facilities (some rural areas even do not have very basic health care elements, such as clean water and preventive vaccines), and most of them do not have any type of health insurance so that they have to pay out of pocket for every medical visit (Chen, 2005). This challenge is both ethically and economically formidable, because the countryside covers about eight hundred million Chinese people, composing about seventy-five percent of the country's entire population.

R. Fan
Department of Public and Social Administration, City University of Hong Kong, Hong Kong, PRC
e-mail: safan@cityu.edu.hk

J. Tao (ed.), *China: Bioethics, Trust, and the Challenge of the Market*,

© Springer Science+Business Media B.V. 2008

3. How should various, multi-level insurance plans be developed to cover most citizens in the cities? The urban medical care insurance scheme recently developed by the government created a new health care model by combining general social insurance and (Singaporean) provident fund arrangements to support health care for urban employees. It has significantly reformed China's past free medical care system (for government employees) and the labor-protection medical care system (for the employees of state-owned enterprises), in which individuals bore no financial obligation for their healthcare and therefore were not seriously concerned with rising healthcare costs (Gao, 2004). However, the scope of this new scheme is quite limited – the employees of private companies and self-employed people are not covered in it. Most unfortunately, it was designed to cover adult employees only, leaving their dependent family members uncovered. This is highly ironic in the context of the Confucian family-oriented cultural values that are still present in China (Fan & Holliday, 2006).
4. What should be done to build a well-ordered health care market? The health care market is rapidly developing in China in meeting the people's multiple, various health needs. But the market is not yet well-ordered (Cao & Wang, 2005). It suffers from a few serious defects:

    1) All state-owned hospitals have been defined as non-profit hospitals, assigned with special privileges to compete for patients and maintain a monopoly in the market. As "non-profit", not only do they not need to pay any tax to the state, but they continuously receive funds from the state. They are insured to get patients because the new urban medical care insurance scheme is generally designed to require its beneficiaries to receive treatments only from such hospitals in order to reimburse their medical costs. Many such hospitals make a huge profit by providing high-tech medical services, including prescribing luxury imported medications, which are not always medically necessary. Consequently, the private sector is hard to compete with them and develop in current China (Du, 2008; Chen, Yang & Shen, 2008). The role of the rising private sector is still marginal in most places, although in a few cities private hospitals have just begun to break the monopoly of the state-owned hospitals. Over the country, there exist only about 1,500 private hospitals, while there are more than 70,000 state-owned hospitals (Chen et al., 2008). Those private hospitals have the merits of relatively low costs, good service attitudes, convenient geographical locations, flexible open times, various methods of payment and sound communication with patients. But they also suffer from small size, unskilled professionals, insufficient facilities and non-qualification for receiving the patients covered by the urban medical care insurance scheme (Chen et al., 2008).
    2) It has not been clearly sorted out what should be an appropriate way for the government to regulate health care markets in general and hospitals in particular. Health care has officially been taken as welfare for the people, and the prices of services have been set low and controlled strictly by the government in the name of adapting people's affordability. Physicians are only allowed to

charge very low fees for their consultations. In order to get payments for their hospitals as well as for themselves, physicians have to "do" something on the patients, such as performing experimental and machinery examinations, procedures, operations, and – most importantly – prescribing drugs to make a profit from the difference between the wholesale prices (at which hospitals purchase drugs from drug companies) and the retail prices (at which hospitals fill the physicians' prescriptions for their patients). Many hospitals could make as much as 50% of their total income from such "selling" of drugs to their patients. This has generally triggered a series of fraudulent medical phenomena, such as over-treatment, over-prescription, prescribing expensive, luxury or imported drugs that are not clearly medically indicated. It has even seduced some physicians to collude with drug companies to prescribe their drugs to patients in order to get kickbacks from the companies (Du, 2008).[2]

5. What should be done to deal with the crisis of trust in health care area? An attitude of distrust is permeating in current Chinese society. Patients suspect that physicians' primary interest is not looking after their health, but to make money; physicians worry that patients would easily find excuses to sue them in order to obtain compensations and thereby engage in protective medicine for their own safety (Li, 2005). Ever-increasing disputes and lawsuits have occurred in health care area. Evidently, this atmosphere of distrust is not limited to the health care area. It is present also in politics, business, education, and in almost every area. It makes the people's ordinary lives unpleasant, general administration and management difficult, and policy and system reforms very hard. With such common distrust, how could the country effectively curb the steady spread of diseases like AIDS, or successfully fight another unexpected epidemic of SARS or Avian Flu? More fundamentally, permeating distrust indicates the corrosion and corruption of the basic moral values and commitments that have been underlying the civil way of Chinese lives. Could China really gain a peaceful rise in the world without seriously reconstructing the Chinese moral values and commitments?

The last point leads us to ethical reflections. Like it or not, our conduct and policy are always affected by our ethic. It is crucially important to tackle these grave challenges facing the Chinese health care from a right moral direction. Of course, a moral reflection does not have to appeal to an ethical principle as a point of departure. Usually real specific and rich moral commitments and values, rather than general principles, are practiced and embodied in the actual way of life in which people are engaged. However, for the sake of moral reflection presented in this paper, I do not have to reject an old cliché in ethics: we cannot appropriately ponder over practical issues without starting from proper ethical principles. Since ethical principles summarize particular ethical practices and provide general ethical orientations, we need to be very careful in selecting a proper set of ethical principles for moral guidance. If we select wrong ethical principles to direct our actions, practical outcomes could be irreversibly damaging. This does not commit us to ethical determinism – it is not that once correct ethical principles are chosen, all practical issues will be automatically resolved. We would still need to work out effective strategies by considering our economic conditions, political realities, institutional facts, and even people's psychological features in order successfully to apply the principles to direct our acts, reshape our systems, and reform our policies. Nevertheless, since different ethical principles point to the very different directions of development, the Chinese must choose a right type of ethical principles to direct their practical agenda in health care.

The next section briefly contends why two influencing ethical perspectives in current China are misleading and improper for guiding policy. It follows by a section that sets out to reconstruct two traditional Confucian ethical principles, ren-yi (humanity-righteousness) and cheng-xin (sincerity and fidelity), that ought to be restored to direct Chinese society. Section 4 turns to the social implications of these Confucian principles, laying out a particular Confucian conception of justice. This is followed by Section 5 that shows how the two Confucians principles shed light on proper ways in which China can handle the health care challenges listed in this introduction. Concluding remarks are covered in the final section.

2 Two Misleading Ethical Views

It is well-known that a modern Western view of morality has been officially adopted in contemporary China. The view remains influential in today's Chinese ethical discussions in general and medical moral explorations in particular. Essentially, it holds that ethical thought is a type of social consciousness, and social consciousness is ultimately determined by social existence. In particular, this view insists, what ethical principles, values, and virtues are accepted and practiced in a society reflects the level of the economic (productive) forces of the society as well as the economic relations and institutions that the people have formed based on the productive forces. In short, according to this view, it is not that people can choose a set of moral principles and values as they see proper and adopt them to guide their acts and shape their social systems. The opposite is more true: morality is shaped, and is continuously reshaped, in terms of changing economic and social realities.

This view is mistaken because it disparages the basic status of morality in human lives. It is true that we cannot create a morality with a robustly new content from nowhere, because we are inevitably affected by a culture or tradition in which we live. But it is totally false to claim that the moral values (such as the moral virtues, specific etiquettes, protocols, rituals, rules and commitments) that we have learned and absorbed from our parents, relatives, neighbors, teachers, and friends are just determined by the economic forces and relations that these people have happened to obtain in their society. The truth is that our moral values have a much stronger and higher spiritual standing than economic factors. For instance, the Confucian moral values of ren (humanity), yi (appropriateness) and xiao (filial piety) have been rooted in the Chinese mind for thousands of years, transcending various types of economic forces and institutions. In addition, this "economically deterministic" view is particularly harmful in a time of social transition and reform: it lures ethical laziness. It fails to encourage people to reshape reality according to their deeply held moral principles, but making them simply surrender to whatever is fashionable in contemporary social tendencies.

Another problem generated by this view is moral disingenuousness. The view assumes that a perfect, selfless, impartial, and egalitarian morality will come into being when each individual is arranged to work for all under a system of public ownership (i.e., all important material assets and properties are stipulated to belong to the public or the state). People have to claim that they hold such a selfless morality in order to show that they are not morally "low" in such an "ideal" society, while at the bottom of their hearts they are more concerned with themselves, their families, relatives, friends, as well as their own institutions. This view blurs out a necessary line between reasonable self-interests and unfair or immoral self-benefits. The results are not a group of individuals created out to work for all "wholeheartedly," but are a great amount of hypocrisy and corruption in the society.

On the other hand, another ethical view has increasingly become fashionable in current China: the liberal social-democratic view. This view engages in an egalitarian ideology and is interested in creating more and more unfounded individual entitlements or rights. Essentially, it claims that every individual have a most extensive set of social, political, and economic rights which must be guaranteed by the state. Under the influence of American philosopher John Rawls' 1971 publication, *A Theory of Justice,* this view has gained a great deal of support from the rising Chinese liberal scholars. Indeed, at first look this view seems appealing because it apparently voices for everyone's interests, in particular for the interests of the week and the poor in a society.

However, it should be recognized that this view leads to grave moral, political and economic hazards. When a welfare entitlement or right is assigned to an individual, society has to take the burden to satisfy him with that right regardless of his moral standing (e.g., whether he is lazy and a voluntary deserving poor). This usually causes free riders in society and is unfair to hard-working individuals and families (Fan, 2002a). Moreover, as Engelhardt indicates, once an entitlement (such as a right to health care) is in the hands of a person, the person and his family will tend to use it to the utmost, even when such use may not be either prudent or cost-effective, because this imposes no further costs on themselves (Engelhardt, 2008). Furthermore, this view tempts politicians to promise benefits to people that will have to be funded by future tax payments, causing long-term political and economic damages (Engelhardt, 2008). Finally, this view is foundationally defective in the moral sense. Since resources are from everyone's work, such unqualified equal entitlements for resources are groundless. Even if it is morally proper or virtuous to help the weak and the poor in society, it does not mean that the justification of the help must be grounded in a system of equal rights or entitlements ensured to everyone by the state. If China applies this view to reform its health care system, the result would be disastrous.

In short, both views are morally misleading and consequently damaging. Neither should be used for guiding Chinese society and health care practices.

3 Reconstructionist Confucian Ethical Principles for Health Care

This section argues that we should reconstruct the Confucian ethical principles to direct our health care system reforms and policy reformulations. Differing from the "economically-deterministic" ethical view, the Reconstructionist Confucianism I am presenting consists of a set of moral principles that are not determined by productive forces, but are mandated by Heaven, rooted in the heart/mind of human beings, articulated by the Confucian sages, and possessing the eternal moral values transcending contemporary society in directing human lives and regulating economic institutions. Unlike the modern Western liberal social-democratic ethical view, Reconstructionist Confucianism is family-oriented rather than individual-centered, junzi-oriented rather than equality-centered, and virtue-oriented rather than rights-centered. It calls for recasting social and economic institutions through reforming public policy in accordance with fundamental Confucian concerns and commitments (Fan, 2002b).

Confucianism should be reconstructed because it has been distorted by various types of anti-Confucian thought and movement in the twentieth century. In the first part of the century, all newly introduced fashionable "isms" – such as Darwinism, positivism, pragmatism, anarchism, Nietzschism, and Marxism – construed Confucianism as a reactionary ideology grounded in China's feudalistic past that should be abandoned as a whole. The notorious slogan "down with the Confucian house" expressed in the May Fourth Movement in 1919 continued to have force throughout the century. The anti-Confucian movement reached its peak in the so-called "Cultural Revolution" in the latter part of the century. The Confucian ethical structures and family commitments as well as the formal Confucian rituals and institutions were ruthlessly insulted and sullied.

Fortunately, Deng Xiaoping's economic reforms woke up many Chinese from their self-damaging cultural nightmares. As the reforms have furthered and deepened, recent Chinese society has witnessed a slow but steady revival of the Confucian values in mainland China. In attempting to reconstruct Confucian ethical principles into a coherent whole to redirect our lives and society, I confess that I am not able to offer a knock-down philosophical argument to show that Confucian ethics is the only proper ethics among competing ethical accounts. As Engelhardt has convincingly shown, the ability of moral epistemology is inevitably limited. We cannot through rational philosophical argument prove any ethical account as canonical without eventually begging the question, arguing in a circle, or engaging infinite regress (Engelhardt, 1996). What I can do is to offer a most complete, least one-sided, and most powerful portrayal of the Confucian insights and reflections on human nature, morality and society so as to expose its ethical authenticity and beauty. The strength of such a Reconstructionist Confucian account is not only from its internal intellectual coherence, but also from its contrasting differences from the "economically deterministic" ethical view and the liberal social-democratic ethical account as well as from its practical implications for directing the market, economy and society in current China.

In particular, I will lay out two fundamental Confucian ethical principles for guiding Chinese health care: the Principle of Ren-Yi (Humanity-Righteousness), and the Principle of Cheng-Xin (Sincerity-Fidelity). Although some modern Western ethical concepts (like "liberty" and "rights") have become fashionable in current Chinese academic discourse, the moral values of ren-yi and cheng-xin are still at home in the ordinary Chinese lives, and these words, rather than the exported "rights" or "liberty," are the ones used in the typical native moral language games. In particular, cheng-xin has recently become one of the most frequently used classical terms, because many feel that cheng-xin is absent in the society in general and in health care area in particular. Many have begun to reconstruct the Confucian virtues of cheng-xin (Li, 2005; Liang et al., 2005; Yang & Wang, 2005; Xu & Chen, 2005; Chen & Lan, 2005) for reshaping the Chinese ethical character in the market. Evidently, in the Confucian tradition ren-yi is a more basic concept than cheng-xin.

3.1 The Principle of Ren-Yi (Humanity-Righteousness)[3]

It is generally agreed that Confucian ethics is a type of virtue ethics. Virtue is not entitlement, but is character required for human flourishing. Confucius (551–479BC) and Mencius (327–289BC) provided a classical Confucian account of virtue based on their understandings of human nature. Humans, for them, are not atomistic, discrete, self-serving individuals coming to construct a society through contract. Humans are by nature familial animals, possessing the potential to form appropriate families and pursue flourishing in familial relations. Confucius identifies ren, the fundamental human virtue, as the quality of "loving humans" (Analects 12:22). Ren has become a most important Confucian ethical ideal. How is loving humans possible? Mencius discloses that Heaven (tian) has endowed the sprout (duan) of ren into everyone's heart/mind: that is, everyone has an innate affection-capacity to love others (Mencius 2A4:3; 2A4:5). However, Mencius also recognizes that one's emotion of love is not equally present for all the people: we naturally love our family members strongly and strangers only weakly. Moreover, even for our relatives, it is often that this feeling of love is able to motivate us only when it is convenient for us to act (Mencius 3A5). Accordingly, in order to fulfill human love, Mencius emphasizes that we must cultivate the sprout of love by extending (tui, ji, da, kuo) it from one context to another and from one person to another (1A7:12; 7A15; 7B31; 2A6), thus developing the feeling into a stable emotional disposition, trait, character, or virtue.

How can one really control one's passion so as to extend love to all humans appropriately? Does Confucianism eventually require loving all humans equally? The answer is no. Confucians do not uphold egalitarian love, neither do they take that sort of love as possible. The appropriate love of humans is, for Confucians, love with distinctions and care by gradation. Indeed, in order to love all humans appropriately, Confucius teaches us to observe rituals (li), a series of ceremonies and rules of propriety (Analects 12:1). Confucius recognizes that only in serious ritual performance can one nurture, manage and control one's emotions. Indeed, if life is like a play, the play must be real in the Confucian ritual participation: Confucius could not bear to see "the forms of mourning conducted without real grief" (Analects 3:26). Instead, one should think of everything one does as participation in ritual: "Behave in public business as though you were in the presence of an important guest. Deal with the people as though you were officiating at an important sacrificial ritual" (Analects 12:2).[4] In short, the seriousness and enjoyability of ritual performance make it possible for one to cultivate a disposition of love for all humans, and different types of ritual make it possible for one to love all humans differently: there are affection (qin) between parent and child, righteousness (yi) between ruler and subject, different function (bie) between husband and wife, order (xu) between old and young, and fidelity (xin) between friend and friend (Mencius 3A4:8).

In short, the fundamental Confucian virtue of ren requires universal love, but not egalitarian love. Love is cultivated and differentiated in performing distinct rituals for different familial and social relationships. In particular, Confucians have advocated transforming such rituals into specific social institutions and policies that are family-oriented and family-friendly (see next section).

Yi is identified by Confucius as another important virtue that junzi, the exemplary person of good character and moral integrity, must possess. First, yi is the character of being able to do what is right (Analects 4:10, 17:23). In this sense it is correct to say that yi is meant appropriateness (Mean 20:5). Second, in order to do what is right, one must not be lured by material benefits to violate moral commitments. Yi is the character that enables one to concentrate on the right in facing benefits (Analects 4:16, 16:10, 19:1). Finally, the best way of practicing yi is honoring the virtuous. If the virtuous is honored in society, their character for doing what is right can be learned and followed by others.[5]

There is an excellent summary of the Confucian virtues of ren and yi in relation to rituals in the Mean:

> Ren is the characteristic element of humanity, and the great exercise of it is in loving relatives. Yi is the accordance with what is appropriate, and the great exercise of it is in honoring the virtuous. The decreasing measure of the love due to relatives, and the steps in the honor due to the worthy, are produced by ritual (Mean 20:5).

This is to say, the major practical requirement of ren is to love relatives (this constitutes the core of Confucian familism), and the major practical requirement of yi is to respect the virtuous (this constitutes the core of Confucian elitism). Both ren and yi are squarely opposed to egalitarian love without distinctions (Fan, 2004). Taken together, the Confucian ethical virtues of ren-yi can generally be summarized as this principle: **family love should be emphasized in practicing universal human love, and the virtuous should be honored in performing what is right**.

3.2 The Principle of Cheng-Xin (Sincerity-Fidelity)

Confucius uses the basic meaning of cheng as "true" or "truly." He claims that it is indeed a cheng (true) saying that "if good men were to govern a country for a hundred years, they would be able to transform the violently bad and dispense with capital punishments" (Analects 12:11). Secondly, in the Great Learning, cheng is emphasized as an attitude of making one's will sincere: this means no self-deception is allowed, and junzi must be watchful over oneself when one is alone (Great Learning 6). Finally, cheng acquires a mystical meaning in the Mean. Here cheng is identified as the way of Heaven, and the attainment of cheng identified as the way of men: it is a sage who is absolutely cheng and therefore can hit upon what is right without effort and apprehend without thinking (Mean 20: 18). It is also characteristic of absolute cheng to be able to foreknow (Mean 24). Cheng is the completion of the self (Mean 25:1). Mencius states that there is no greater delight than to be conscious of cheng on self-examination (Mencius 7A:4). In short, cheng is the deep moral character of the Confucian embodied in the most sincere, serious and complete commitments to the ren-yi. In this regard, cheng is not only a state of mind, but is also an active spiritual force that can complete humans and draw them and Heaven together into a unity.

The basic meaning of xin is that one is careful about one's words, not using them to deceive others, and that one must mean what one says and seriously keeps one's words and promises (Analects 1:5, 1:6, 1:7, 1:8, 1:13, 2:22). Moreover, xin carries a more positive sense in that one (especially a leader) must be faithfully dedicated to the wellbeing of those one is engaging so as to gain their trust (Analects 5:26, 12:7; Mencius 3A4: 8; Great Learning 3, 10; Mean 20:14, 20:17, 29:2, 31:3, 33:3). This is to say, honesty and loyalty are taken to be the conditions of trust that Confucianism wants to promote in society.

Taken together, the Confucian ethical virtues of cheng-xin can generally be summarized as this principle: **moral sincerity should be promoted, maintaining the unity of one's words and acts, and being trustworthy in dealings with others**.

Needless to say, these two principles are by no means exhaustive of important Confucian ethical principles. However, if my account is sound, they carry significant moral implications for a proper view of social justice as well as for reforming and reshaping health care institutions and policies.

4 Implications for Social Justice

The Confucian account of social justice based on these two principles would be sharply different from either the "economically deterministic" account or the liberal social-democratic account (Fan, 2003a). First, Confucians support an economic system in which people own private property, rather than a system that only permits state or public ownership. This is because, as Mencius argues, government cannot manifest any love of people if people are deprived of private property:

> The way of the people is this: if they have private property (heng-chan), they will have a fixed heart; if they do not have private property, they will not have a fixed heart. And if they do not have a fixed heart, there is nothing they will not do in the way of self-abandonment, moral deflection, depravity, and wild license. When they have thus involved in crime, to

> follow them up and punish them is to entrap them. How can such a thing as entrapping the people be done under the rule of a ren man? (Mencius 3A3: 3).[6]

There might be some perfect persons, on the Confucian view, who can wholeheartedly work for others without seeking any private property. But that is not the case for ordinary people. The Chinese experience of the "big pot" system in the twentieth century convincingly proves Mencius' observation. To avoid the moral disaster of "entrapping people," the Confucian principle of ren-yi requires the establishment of a private economy.

Second, the market is a morally and economically inevitable mechanism for mediating the interactions among individuals, families, and communities. Frederic Fransen, in his paper for this conference, has succinctly explained why it is a misunderstanding that the interests of consumers could be better realized if a central authority controlled the prices in markets (Fransen, 2008). Complicated economic information must be handled directly by consumers in the market in order to satisfy and adjust their desires. Confucians have shared this wisdom. For instance, Mencius argues, not only do people naturally work on different things and need to exchange them in markets, it is also that different things have unequal quality and it would only cause confusion to control prices by government:

> It is the nature of things to be of unequal quality. Some are worth twice or five times, ten or a hundred times, even a thousand or ten thousand times, more than others. If you reduce them to the same level, it will only bring confusion to the world. If a roughly finished shoe sells at the same price as a finely finished one, who would make the latter? If we follow that way..., we will be showing one another the way to being dishonest (Mencius 3A4: 18).

The appropriate role of government is not to control prices, but is to maintain the order of the market according to the Confucian principle of cheng-xin so that the market can become a system of honest and trust in which individuals and families can effectively exchange benefits.[7]

Thirdly, families are the basic social units for taking care of their members' welfare and bearing financial responsibilities. Confucianism understands that individuals are naturally born to, grow in, and cared by families. The virtue of ren encourages parents to work hard – and save money in particular – for their children's development and welfare. Adult children should be filial to their parents and take care of them when they become elderly.[8] Confucians generally support family-based opportunities even if they are unequal among families. They do not want state-imposed egalitarian opportunities because they have to violate the autonomy of the family – for instance, Confucian families take it as their natural duty to decide investing more resources to their children's education as they see fit. Accordingly, Confucians insist that resources must be left to families for taking care of their members' welfare. For instance, Mencius argues that "a government of ren ... must make the taxes and levies light" (Mencius 1A5:3).[9] Confucius took the heavy taxes and levies as worse than aggressive wild beasts that attacked human lives.

Finally, the principle of ren-yi supports the assistance of the weak and poor in society by a family-centered, virtue-sensitive, non-egalitarian policy. Such assistance should be offered not based on a consideration that creates egalitarian individual entitlements or rights – it is not the Confucian view that every individual is entitled to be ensured by the state with a level of welfare equal to everyone else (Fan, 2003b). Rather, assistance should be offered based on the virtues of ren and yi grounded in a natural sympathy or love. Traditional Confucian scholars argue that government should take limited acts in supporting specially weak groups of people, such as (1) those who do not have complete families, like widows, widowers, orphans, and the childless, (2) the handicapped, and (3) those who encounter unusual natural disasters (like flood and famine). This is to say, state aid can only serve as an unusual rescue method and cannot become usual means for life – the usual, normal help must be from the family. An egalitarian welfare system based on equal rights or entitlements is in tension with the Confucian virtues of ren-yi, because ren requires family-oriented love and responsibility, and yi requires honoring the worthy and hard workers, without awarding the lazy.

5 Health Care Policy Reforms

What does all this mean to the five challenges we have listed in the first section? This section offers certain basic ideas to approach them in accordance with the Confucian principles of ren-yi and cheng-xin.

1. To build a sustainable health care system for the heavily populated Chinese society with an ever increasing portion of the retired elderly, the first important issue is to clarify who bears primary financial responsibility for health care. If the answer is, as the liberal social-democratic view suggests, that the state must through taxation ensure every individual to receive a basic health care package (according to needs) equal to anyone else in the society regardless of their financial situations, then a Chinese health care system thus established would definitely be unsustainable. The reason is evident. First, the huge public investments required by such a system are infeasible for current China, remaining a poor developing country in considering its average GDP per capita. Second, even if such a system can be set up by imposing high taxation, its ever-souring economic burden will destroy the contrary's economic development, which in turn makes the system unsustainable, not to mention the administrative costs, likely corruptions and other types of moral, political and social hazards that must involve in running such a system.

In addition to this economic consideration, the Confucian principle of ren-yi does not advocate such a system on the moral ground. As indicated, Confucianism views welfare financing (including health care payment) as a family responsibility, rather than a state responsibility. Chinese families must save resources by themselves, rather than rely on the state, to support their family members' health care. Strategically, China can learn a great deal from the Singaporean family-saving-based Central Provident Fund system for social security in general and its Medisave plan for health care in particular. That is, it is basically every family's obligation to save resources in order to take care of their members' health care. Of course, families do not have to pay for medical services directly out of their savings accounts. They can use their savings to purchase health insurance plans as they see fit. It is the basic obligation of the government to help create and maintain a well-ordered health care market according to the Confucian principle of cheng-xin. Once such a market is developed, it naturally supplies various types of health insurance plans (with distinct quantities and qualities of benefits promised based on different premium and co-payment requirements) for families to select.

No doubt, this family-responsibility-based health care system would involve unequal enjoyments of health care among families. But it should be recognized that no health care system can result in an equal outcome for everyone, because that equality is practically impossible. Even the theoretically strict egalitarian health care system of Canada cannot prevent its rich families from flying to the United States for quicker or better medical services (Iltis, 2008). The family-oriented system that the Confucian principle of ren-yi supports has the merit of directing and leaving resources to families for efficient uses in the market, without being taxed heavily by government. To maintain the vitality of family responsibilities, the government's health care aid should only be offered to very special groups of people, such as orphans, who do not have families to rely on, or in very special cases in which the families encounter unavoidable difficulties. The government aids offered in the latter cases must be short-term rescue methods rather than long-term welfare projects. Public resources, if available, should primarily spent in promoting general goods for public health, such as providing health education, improving the environment, and offering preventive vaccines.

The success of such a family-oriented health care system will eventually depend on the extent to which Chinese families will flourish and maintain their Confucian ethical features, such as ren and xiao. It is high time for the Chinese government to reconsider its "one child per couple" policy. The policy is not only culturally damaging, but is also economically costing. In the long run how China would not be able to support a huge amount of the elderly when there are no sufficient youths in the workforce.

2. The health care challenges from the countryside should be heart-broken to all Chinese, especially those in the government. It is certainly true that the government invested much less health care resources in the countryside than in cities. But the more striking truth is that the government levies much higher tax rates on rural families than on urban families, even when the average income of rural families is significantly lower than that of urban families. It is urgently important for the government to improve and regulate itself by following the Confucian principles of ren-yi and cheng-xin. Following these principles, the first crucial thing to do is to reform the unfair system of taxation for the countryside and get rid of various unreasonable fees imposed on the peasants (the government has recently rightly cancelled the agricultural tax, but this is far from being enough). How well this can be done depends on how well the government can shrink the size of itself – especially at its local levels in the countryside – and improve its management. And this eventually depends on how sincere the government officials are willing to follow the Confucian principles of ren-yi and cheng-xin.

The current government trial of setting up a cooperative medical insurance plan for the peasants (especially for those in impoverished places) shows a good intention. But occurring problems indicate how important it is for the government to comply with the principle of cheng-xin in its governance. First, according to the design of this plan, for the total premium of RMB$30 for a peasant's annual health insurance, $10 is from the peasant, $10 is from the central government, and $10 is from a local government. But many local governments complain that they do not have the money – or they can afford the money in the first year as a special political obligation but not for following years. Second, many peasants do not want to join the plan because they do not trust its reliability. Finally, some peasants who already joined the plan had difficulties in seeking the benefits (especially reimbursements) as originally promised so that they want to withdraw from it (Chen, 2005). All this shows that this government-initiated and government-running insurance plan, although being a very low-level, minimal insurance (rightly being so), is not very promising to become a stable health plan for most rural areas. It is high time for the government to consider changing its role as a provider to a role of regulator. If the government could help create and maintain a well-ordered market in the countryside, various types of private insurance plans will emerge for peasants to choose.

3. The recently developed urban medical care insurance scheme run by the government should be reformed to make it a family-based scheme – that is, all family members should be covered so as to manifest the Confucian virtue of ren-yi. Moreover, the government should not manage to make this scheme become the only dominant insurance plan in urban areas. A more appropriate work for the government is to create an environment in which various reliable insurance plans can be worked out and exist so that families can select according to their particular needs and expectations.

4. Everyone sees a big health care market in China. But the market is not appropriately operated yet. Indeed, there are two misleading views on the market in current China. One view is that it is good to kick away any morality so as to use the market to maximize profits. The other view is that the development of the market must be curbed or limited by the government because profit-making in the market necessarily causes moral problems. Both views overlook the moral values underlying the necessary condition of the market. The necessary condition of the market is trust: if people do not have mutual trust, market transactions would be impossible. It is the very virtues of cheng-xin (sincerity-fidelity) possessed by individuals that make mutual trust possible. So the real issue is not for the government to curb the development of the market, but is to maintain the order of the market. It is going to be a great task for the Chinese government to learn and become a good order-maintainer, rather than a profit-pursuer, of the market.

(a) I agree with Professor Du Zhizheng that the government should break down the monopolistic position of the state-owned, "non-profit" hospitals by re-identifying them (Du, 2008). Most of them should be privatized and defined as for-profit hospitals so that they should pay profit tax to the government. At the same time they should gain freedom to decide their service prices as well as their preferred targets of patients. The rest hospitals, remaining state-owned and non-profit, should receive more funds from the government to support their staff and services. The targets of their patients should be those from middle- and low-income families who do not have a first-rate health insurance or have to pay out of pocket, and the prices of their services should be monitored by the government. In this way it is hopeful to form a healthy competitive environment between private and public hospitals.

(b) The development of private hospitals should be encouraged rather than curbed (Chen et al., 2008). Private and foreign capitals should all be allowed to invest in Chinese health care. A fair competition between private and public hospitals is the effective way of pushing them to improve their services as well as curbing the unreasonable rising of health care costs, as long as the government could maintain the order of the market. At this point (before various health insurance plans are available in Chinese society), it is a very good suggestion that the government-run urban health insurance scheme should not limit its beneficiaries only to state-owned hospitals. Private hospitals should receive a fair chance for competition (Chen et al., 2008).

(c) Even if the government is in the position of supervising the state-owned, public hospitals and monitoring their service prices, it is not wise for the government to keep a very low consultation fees for physicians to charge. Medical professional knowledge and practical wisdom do not have to be manifested in offering machinery examinations or operations, much less in the value of drug selling. A right judgment or a wise advice offered to a patient is often crucial to that patient's health. The time and energy that the physician invests in such consultation should be appropriately respected through a reasonable price. In that case the physician would not have to "embody" his value in prescribing expensive drugs in order to gain an income.[10]

5. Finally, what else can we say and do about the crisis of trust? It is clear that the important task is not simply to call for more trust, but is to build necessary conditions for trust. As Ana Iltis shows, moral integrity is a necessary condition for trust (Iltis, 2008). If we fail to cultivate integrity, we cannot achieve trust in society. The Confucian moral integrity is cheng-xin (sincerity-fidelity). This involves a serious reconstruction of the Confucian moral virtues at the levels of the government, institution, and individual. At the level of the government, officials should sincerely hold the virtues of caring the people and honoring the worthy, honestly recognize that the best way of benefiting the people is creating a well-ordered market rather than carrying out centrally planned and controlled comprehensive plans, and seriously become a regulator (rather a player) of the market. At the level of institution, it is important to establish commitments and determine their implications for organizational life: will the organization be a secular or belief-based organization? What type of patients will be cared for? What will be the role of profit for the organization? Finally, individual physicians should recognize that the virtues if ren-yi and cheng-xin are rewarding. Honestly treating others can gain trust and respect for oneself. Eventually, sincere, trustworthy and wise moral conduct is most pleasant in life.

6 Concluding Remarks

The health care challenges facing China are enormous. But a more fundamental challenge is for the Chinese to reconstruct their moral and cultural commitments. Chinese people are gradually abandoning the instrumentalist, "economically deterministic" view of morality. The danger of the liberal social-democratic morality looms large. As Engelhardt reminds us, in order to fashion a sustainable health care financing scheme, an entitlement mentality as well as an egalitarian ideology must be avoided (Engelhardt, 2008). This paper argues that the best we can do is to reconstruct the Confucian virtues of ren-yi and cheng-xin so as to build a family-based and virtue-oriented Chinese health care system.

Notes

1 See Engelhardt's paper for this conference. It seems that many Chinese scholars have been "occupied" by some other "current" issues and have not clearly recognized this "long-term" difficulty facing the Chinese in affording health care.

2 Restricting physicians charging from consultations is a significant moral and economic issue. To my disappointment, I have not found much discussion in the Chinese literature on this issue. From my personal experience, Chinese physicians often complain that they cannot make any money from consultation, no matter how knowledgeable, skillful, and experienced they are. They are "forced" to sell drugs to get an income.

2 There are many different English translations of ren and yi. Some may want to translate ren as "benevolence" and yi as "justice" so that the Confucian principle becomes the principles of benevolence and justice. Since the Confucian vision of ren and yi is dramatically different from the liberal social-democratic account of benevolence and justice (e.g., that offered through Tom Beauchamp and James Childress' mid-level bioethical principles), I don't choose these English words for ren and yi. All my citations of the Confucian classics are adapted translations of my own based on James Legge (1970, 1971).

4 I have followed David Nivision's excellent explanation on this issue. See Nivision (1996, p. 105).

5 Mencius explains that everyone has a basic hear/mind of shame and dislike that makes honoring the virtuous possible.

6 It is a big misunderstanding that (1) the market economy based on private ownership did not occur in China until it was imported from the modern Western economic system, and (2) that Confucianism traditionally did not support private ownership and the market. Neither is true. As a solid and careful research made by Zhao Gang and Chen Zhongyi shows, the Chinese system of private ownership already formed in the Warring-Sate Period of China – more than two thousand years ago. Confucians before Mencius may have supported a public-ownership system – the Well-field System of Land – most of them no longer did so since Mencius. Instead, as Zhao and Chen indicate, Mencius call for "forming property for the people" (wei min zhi chan) helped to bring about the privatization of land (See Zhao & Chen, 1991, p. 5).

7 The Confucian advocacy of a market economy based on privately-owned and privately-run businesses is vividly illustrated in a famous book, *The Debate on Salt and Iron* (written in 81, B.C.), recording a debate between Confucian scholars and Legalist officials regarding the economic institutions and fiscal measures adopted at the time. The Legalist officials supported government monopolies in the contemporary vital industries of salt, iron, liquor, coinage, and government trading. They argued that the government control of these industries was necessary to ensure government revenues and to maintain defensive warfare against the *xun-nu* tribes who threatened the empire. Also, according to these Legalists, by owning and running these industries directly, the government could protect people from exploitation by private businessmen and corporations. On the other hand, the Confucian

scholars argued that China should make peace with other nations and should not grasp the land of its neighbors. Moreover, they pointed to the fact that, contrary to the argument of the Legalists, it was the corruption and maladministration in the government system of monopolies that were forcing people to use the inferior products of salt and iron and at times to do without them entirely. In short, these Confucian scholars argued that the people should have a right to use natural resources to benefit themselves, while government should never make material profit as a motive of its administration so as to compete with people in pursuing profits. For an excellent English abstract of this book, see De Bary, et al. (1960, pp. 218–223). For Neo-Confucianism in shaping and supporting a modern Chinese business ethics (especially the virtues of industry, frugality, and cheng-xin), see Yu, 1996.

8 Following the Confucian familist morality, it remains a legal duty of married children to take care of elderly parents in need. Such duty is stipulated in the Chinese Marriage Law in mainland China.

9 Confucians usually argue that the government tax rates should be no more than 10 percent of a family's income. See *Analects 12.9.*

10 I am not saying that once the government loosens or cancels the restriction on this, over-prescription and other types of physician corruption will automatically disappear. But that restriction is no doubt a significant psychological and economic inducer. Morally, we don't have any good reason to obliterate the value of physician's professional training, knowledge, and wisdom that are manifested in their consultations with patients.

References

Cao, Y., & Wang, Y. (2005). The effect of the Chinese health care market on the physician-patient relation. *Medicine and Philosophy* (yixue yu zhexue), *26*(2), 9–11.

Chen, Y. (2005). New cooperative medical care system in the countryside and the humanist concerns with peasants' health. *Chinese Medical Ethics* (Zhongguo yixue lunlixue), *18*(2), 73–75.

Chen, L., & Lan, Y. (2005). Cheng-xin education and medical virtue construction. *Chinese Medical Ethics* (Zhongguo yixue lunlixue), *18*(1), 11–13.

Chen, X., Yang, T., & Shen, X. (2008). Medical resources, markets and the development of private hospitals in China, In J. Tao (ed.), *China: Bioethics, Trust, and the Challenge of the Market,* Springer, pp. 45–54.

Confucius. (1971). *Confucian analects, the great learning and the doctrine of the mean.* J. Legge Trans.). New York: Dover Publications, Inc.

De Bary, W.T., Chan, W., & Watson, B. (Eds.) (1960). *Sources of Chinese tradition* (Vol. 1). New York: Columbia University Press.

Du, Z. (2008). Health care services, markets, and the Confucian moral tradition, establishing a humanistic health care market, In J. Tao (ed.), *China: Bioethics, Trust, and the Challenge of the Market,* Springer, pp. 137–150.

Engelhardt, H. T., Jr. (1996). *The foundations of bioethics* (2nd ed.). New York: Oxford University Press.

Engelhardt, H. T., Jr. (2008). China, Beware: What American health care has to learn from Singapore, In J. Tao (ed.), *China: Bioethics, Trust, and the Challenge of the Market,* Springer, pp. 55–71.

Fan, R. (2002a). Health care allocation and the Confucian tradition. In X. Jang (Ed.), *The examined life - Chinese perspectives: Vol. 1. Association of Chinese Philosophers, in America (ACPA) series of Chinese and Comparative Philosophy* (pp. 211–233). Binghamton, New York: Global Publications.

Fan, R. (2002b). Reconstructionist Confucianism and bioethics, a note on moral difference. In H. T. Engelhardt, Jr. & L. Rasmussen (Eds.), *Bioethics and moral content, national traditions of health care morality* (pp. 281–287). Dordrecht: Kluwer Academic Publishers.

Fan, R. (2003a). Social justice, rawlsian or Confucian?. In B. Mou (Ed.), *Comparative approaches to Chinese philosophy* (pp. 144–168). UK: Ashgate Publishing Ltd.

Fan, R. (2003b). Rights or Virtues? Toward a reconstructionist Confucian bioethics. In R. Qiu (Ed.), *Bioethics, Asian perspectives* (pp. 57–68). Dordrecht: Kluwer Academic Publishers.

Fan, R. (2004). Is a Confucian family-oriented civil society possible? In D. A. Bell & C. Hahm (Eds.), *The politics of affective relations, East Asia and beyond* (pp. 75–96). Oxford: Lexington Books.

Fan, R., & Holliday, I. (2006). Comparative healthcare system models in East Asia. In G. M. Leung & J. Bacon-Shone (Eds.), *Hong Kong's health system, reflections, perspectives and visions.* University of Hong Kong Press, 95–107.

Fransen, F. (2008). Markets, trust, and the nurturing of a culture of responsibility, implications for health care policy, In J. Tao (ed.), *China: Bioethics, Trust, and the Challenge of the Market,* Springer, pp. 151–168.

Gao, J. (2004). On the necessity of perfecting the Chinese health security system in the transitional stage. *Medicine and Philosophy* (yixue yu zhexue), *25*(12), 47–48.

Iltis, A. (2008). The Pursuit of an efficient, sustainable health care system in China, In J. Tao (ed.), *China: Bioethics, Trust, and the Challenge of the Market,* Springer, pp. 89–116.

Li, B. (2008). Trust is the core of the Doctor–patient relationship, from the viewpoint of traditional Chinese medical ethics, In J. Tao (ed.), *China: Bioethics, Trust, and the Challenge of the Market,* Springer, pp. 39–44.

Li, S. (2005). Physician–patient conflict and the absence of trust. *Medicine and Philosophy* (yixue yu zhexue), *25*(3), 25–27.

Liang, H., Guo, Z., Li, G., & Min, J. (2005). Cheng-xin should become an important category in modern medical ethical theory. *Chinese Medical Ethics* (Zhongguo yixue lunlixue), *18*(1), 1–4.

Mencius (1970). *The works of Mencius.* J. Legge (Trans.). New York: Dover Publications, Inc.

Nivision, D. (1996). *The ways of Confucianism.* Chicago: Open Court.

Xu, N., & Chen, X. (2005). The moral defects in current medical advertisements and ethical reconstruction. *Chinese Medical Ethics* (Zhongguo yixue lunlixue), *18*(1), 8–10.

Yang, T., & Wang, Y. (2005). Cheng-xin, from virtues and utilities to responsibilities and rights. *Chinese Medical Ethics* (Zhongguo yixue lunlixue), *18*(1), 5–7.

Yu, Y. (1996). *Chinese modern religious ethics and the spirit of businessman* (Zhongguo Jingshi Zhongjiao Lunli yu Shangren Jingsheng). Taiwan: Lianjing.

Zhao, G., & Chen, Z. (1991). *A history of Chinese economic systems* (Zhongguo Jinji Zhidushi). Beijing: Chinese Economic Press.

Part IV
The Market and Health Care

Health Care Services, Markets, and the Confucian Moral Tradition: Establishing a Humanistic Health Care Market

Zhizheng Du

1 Introduction

Today, the disease structure has changed, the number of elderly people has increased, and high-tech medicine is now widely used. All of these factors have increased the costs of healthcare. Because the government cannot provide free healthcare for everyone, market mechanisms have to be introduced into the healthcare system. Governments, which originally provided free medical services, are now introducing market mechanisms into the healthcare system. Healthcare is a basic right, and both the supply and demand sectors of the healthcare system have their own unique characteristics. Medical services should not be purchased through the market like other market commodities. China like many governments, which introduced market mechanisms into their healthcare systems, is facing a good deal of problems. One way to solve these problems is to establish a unique healthcare system according to market regulation rules in order to minimize negative effects; another way is to appeal to traditional Chinese moral principles to account for the flaws in market mechanisms. We can establish healthcare service markets, which conform to human nature.

2 The Four Stages of Chinese Healthcare Reform

China's healthcare system has been changing ever since China began to carry out its policy of reform and "opening-up" in the 1980s (Annals of China's Health, 1990, pp. 8–10). China has been reforming its healthcare system for nearly two decades. The reform efforts have focused on how the healthcare system can adapt to the market economic environment and how it can make use of some market mechanisms to enhance the vitality of the healthcare industry to better satisfy the people's demands for healthcare. However, some problems have arisen in the process. The market for some hospitals in some areas is bigger, while in other areas, it is

---

Z. Du
Dalian Medical University, PRC
e-mail: duzhi@mail.dlptt.ln.cn

J. Tao (ed.), *China: Bioethics, Trust, and the Challenge of the Market*,
© Springer Science+Business Media B.V. 2008

smaller. Although more than 10 years of experience has helped us to understand the relationship between healthcare and the market, we have not reached unanimity until now. Generally speaking, unlike the public, the majority of hospital managers and employees welcomed the marketing and commercialization of healthcare services.

2.1 The First Stage: 1987–1990

In 1987, the State Council decided to introduce a contracted management system to large and medium sized enterprises, to provide an added impetus for health services. This began with sample experiments to determine whether a contracted system would be successful. Thereafter, a handful of provinces began to implement planned experiments. This contracted system was to introduce the operating mechanisms of the market economy to heath care so hospitals could be self-managing, responsible for profits and losses, and have self-renewing commodity management. That was the first step of healthcare reform in China. Introducing a contracted management system improved the efficiency of healthcare services and increased the vitality and profits of hospitals within a certain period of time. However, there were a few hospitals that only wanted to earn money and make profits while having neglected patients, which aroused strong protests from all classes of society. As a result, health services suspended this simple contracted responsibility system in 1990, and emphasized that hospitals should make it a priority to benefit society and carry out reforms, which stressed equally both economic profits and societal benefits (Annals of China's Health, 1990, pp. 8–10).

2.2 The Second Stage: 1990–1997

The second round of China's reform of the healthcare system began in 1990 (Annals of China's Health, 1991, pp. 3–5). This reform effort focused on how to establish an administrative system and a market-compatible micro-operation system in a health organization, according to the demands of the market economy and healthcare laws. The goal was to guarantee people's basic healthcare needs, to correctly control the application range and power of both planned and market regulations to unite them together, to reform the administration and service systems in the healthcare system, and to reasonably arrange and distribute health resources and develop their maximum profit potential. Specialist clinics and wards, nominated operations, high quality services for high prices and priority for high prices appeared during this period of reform. The main objective of this round of reforms was to explore how to combine planned regulations with market regulations (Annals of China's Health, 1992, pp. 8–11).

2.3 The Third Stage: 1997–2003

In 1997, the Chinese Communist Party and Chinese government decided to reform and develop China's healthcare system (Annals of China's Health, 1998, pp. 3–5).

In 1998, the State Council decided to establish a basic medical insurance system for urban employees (Annals of China's Health, 1999, pp. 3–4), and in 1999 the State Council's eight committees and the Country's System Reform Committee, decided to reform the urban healthcare system (Annals of China's Health, 2000, pp. 3–6), which initiated the third step of China's healthcare reform. This measure was based on the recognition that the healthcare system is a public welfare facility with certain social welfare functions, which everybody needs and benefits from. The goals were as follows: to build up a market-compatible urban healthcare system, to promote the development of healthcare organizations and medical industries and to make sure that people could enjoy reasonably-priced, good quality medical service, and to improve the status of people's health. The essence of this step was to combine planned regulations with market regulations by the following: (1) classifying hospitals into profit-making ones and non-profit ones, (2) establishing and perfecting the healthcare system so that community healthcare organizations, comprehensive hospitals and specialized hospitals could properly assign their work, (3) implementing regional healthcare projects and strengthening the general modulation of healthcare resources, (4) expanding the decision-making power of state-owned hospitals, and building up their internal inspiration and restriction mechanisms, (5) creating a separate branch for the management of medical services and drugs, (6) adjusting the prices of medical services by allowing non-profit hospitals to have control over incomes, price management and restructuring and permitting free prices in profit-making hospitals, (7) implementing a social medical insurance system, where both personal contributions and overall social arrangements are combined and guarantee the basic medical requirements of employees, while taking into account the financial capacities of industries and individuals (The money paid by the employees themselves came from their personal account, while 30% of the costs were paid by the factories where the employees worked. The other 70% of the money was put in an overall arrangements' fund), (8) marking up the upper level and the lower level of the sum of money paid from the overall arrangements' fund. The lower level was about 10% of the average salary of the local employees and the upper level was four times the average salary. The expenses below the lower level should be paid from the personal account or be paid by the individuals themselves. The expenses between the lower level and the upper level were to be paid from the overall arrangements' funds, but workers also needed to pay a certain sum. The expenses above the upper level were paid for by commercial medical insurance. Presently, China is still implementing and perfecting these measures.

2.4 The Fourth Stage: 2004–Present

The target of this stage is to continue implementing the measures recommended in the preceding stage and to provide for better management regulations, convenient healthcare services, and reasonable prices for healthcare services (Annals of China's Health, 2001).

Efforts were made to reform the healthcare system in China because the country did not have the ability to satisfy the ever-increasing objective requirements of health service with the revenue that it was receiving and because the interests of those working in the healthcare industry services needed to be addressed (for example, the improvement of hospitals' management conditions and the promotion of the salaries and welfare of their employees) was an important impetus for the reform of healthcare (Cao & Fu, 2005).

3 The Effects of Healthcare Reform

Reviewing the practices of China's reform, which began in the mid-1980s, the following were achieved (Lu & Zhou, 1993, pp. 9–11; Han & Cheng, 1996, pp. 24–25; Ge, 2005):

(1) Hospitals introduced some market mechanisms and began to practice self-management. They enjoyed sufficient decision-making power in the design of their service items. They also had control of their scales, and could make decisions regarding employees and the purchase of their facilities. Therefore, they had greatly improved the enthusiasm of hospital managers and aided in the development of healthcare. Also, without increasing the country's investments, many hospitals had improved the number of sickbeds, the scale of hospitals and the condition of the environment of the hospitals.
(2) The healthcare services were able to satisfy the special requirements of healthcare consumers. After the reform, special clinics, sickrooms, and services satisfied the different demands for healthcare services.
(3) After market mechanisms were introduced to hospitals and the incomes of medical personnel were directly linked with their work, the enthusiasm of hospital managers and employees had been mobilized and they were able to realize their potentials. And without increasing the number of employees, many hospitals had increased the number of sickbeds and opened specialist clinics, special wards and other special services, which satisfied different people's different healthcare needs and the income of medical personnel greatly increased.
(4) The hospitals had overcome the disadvantage that everything should be done according to the country's orders, which incited the enthusiasm of the hospital managers to employ new techniques. More and more hospitals purchased new types of equipment, adopted new techniques and attracted talents of high level. Because China's rural hospitals, especially some large to medium sized hospitals increased their number of advanced equipment and high and new technologies, they made substantial progress in their level of medical care.

However, the marketing and commercializing of healthcare services also led to some negative consequences (Ran, 2005):

(1) Introducing market mechanisms to healthcare impelled hospitals to pursue profits and deviate from their real objectives. The introduction of market

mechanisms was mainly the introduction of a competition mechanism, a managed account mechanism and a free fluctuation mechanism. Moreover, all of these mechanisms were driven by the pursuit of profits. The pursuit of profits had an effect on the control of the scales of hospitals, the choice of medical equipment, the establishment of service items and the operation of prices. Hospitals "recognized money instead of people" and sick people without money could not get into hospitals. Consequently, this resulted in better healthcare for rich people. People whose income was relatively low, and who could not pay for the costs of medical treatment were deprived of their rights to healthcare. Occasionally, patients who had no money were rejected by hospitals (Xinghua News Agency, 2001).

(2) The commercialization of healthcare brought about a drastic rise of medical expenditures, which burdened not only the country, but also enterprises as well as individuals. People's access to medical treatment was influenced by these increases in cost. Because hospitals regarded pursuing profits as their objective, many hospitals expanded the range of charges, misused new techniques and expensive drugs, prolonged the time patients spent in hospitals and expanded the indications of operations. This resulted in a great increase in medical expenditures, and, in turn, resulted in the increase in the amount of payments made by the country, enterprises, and the individuals (Du, W., 2000; Qing, 2000).

(3) The commercialization of healthcare brought about the waste and inequitable distribution of medical resources. Because the hospitals regarded pursuing profits as their objective, they bought new equipment, employed advanced technology, and imported drugs in large quantities, without consideration of the practical requirements. As a result, a great deal of medical resources (including talent, equipments and funds) were used by larger hospitals and medical centers. These hospitals, in turn, would misuse this new equipment in order to earn back the cost and gain further profits, without considering when they were necessary for treating the patient. It also resulted in a serious imbalance of the distribution of medical resources between cities and villages, primary hospitals and large-medium sized hospitals, developed areas and remote areas (Guo & Du, 2002, pp. 47–49; Zhao, 2000, pp. 7–10).

(4) The commercialization of healthcare weakened prophylaxis and primary healthcare. Because prophylaxis and primary healthcare couldn't bring hospitals or prophylactic organizations big profits, their work was severely crippled since market mechanisms were introduced to the healthcare system. In these organizations, technicians could not be supplemented, and because the funds were diminishing, they didn't have the money to buy equipment and their structures shrank. The public health and primary health care situation were getting worse and worse, and the overall level of the country's healthcare declined (Ge, 2005).

(5) The marketing and commercialization of healthcare services triggered corruption. A few hospital administrators and employees carelessly diagnosed and treated patients. The number of medical accidents and disputes rose rapidly. A handful of medical employees took "red packs" (a kind of bribe sent by patients), or even asked patients for them (Li, 1993, pp. 77–78). A few other

medical employees colluded with drug salesmen and received kickbacks from their malpractice of prescription rights. A minority of the medical employees privately transferred patients to other hospitals or illegally worked for other for-profit hospitals (Fan, 1999, pp. 17–18; Da, 1999, pp. 12–13).

4 Establishing Humanitarian Market Orders for Healthcare Services

Many economists believe that the market is not the solution to every problem (He, 2005). Some economists pay attention to the negative effects of the market. Regulating medical healthcare services according to the market is not an ideal choice. It is a choice that we have to choose. Many problems are inevitable because of general market operations, but many of these problems come from non-standard and distorted market operations. Because of various reasons, it is impossible to prevent market mechanisms from entering the healthcare system completely. We have to establish a healthcare market that conforms to human beings. This kind of market is called an accurate market or an inferior market. According to this model, the objective of hospitals is to treat illnesses and to save the life of the patient; it is not to create the profit. This is the basic difference between a hospital and a commercial enterprise. The hospital is a welfare institution by its nature. Today, the hospital cannot be merely a charitable organization; however, we cannot turn the hospital into a commercial enterprise just because it has adopted market mechanisms (Du, Z., 1991, pp. 296–298; Wang, 1993, pp. 67–69).

Now because the basic objective of healthcare is to prevent disease, treat illnesses, serve people's health, when the contradiction between seeking profit and treating illness occurs, treating illness should be the priority. A hospital cannot stop treatment just because it cannot make money.

What kind of roles does a hospital play in society? The social responsibility of a hospital is to maintain people's health in order to benefit our society. The hospital is not responsible for providing money for the government. A hospital has the following duties: to provide healthcare for the people, promoting fair healthcare, to build public health institutions, to defend patient's rights and to protect the environment. Right now, many hospitals are not adhering to these duties.

The fact that a market mechanism was introduced into hospital management does not mean we can run a hospital just like we would an enterprise. When market mechanisms were introduced into the healthcare system, hospitals are only allowed to use some market rules to improve the management of hospitals; the nature and the objective of the hospital does not change. The objective of the hospital always has priority. The effort to reform hospital management in our country has failed because people have ignored the difference between running hospitals and running enterprises. It should be clear that there are limits to marketing medical services. Applying market management rules to medical services does not mean that all healthcare services are products in the market. We must differentiate between those healthcare services that are allowed to enter the market and those that are not allowed to enter the market. Those healthcare services that are allowed to enter the market are:

(1) Healthcare services, which are not considered basic healthcare.
(2) Special demands (for example, requesting a single hospital ward or high-level service hospital ward).
(3) Special services, such as reproduction technology, kidney transplantation, kidney dialysis and so on.
(4) The non-urgent special services used to rescue life.

In this field, the market should determine the price of the service, the government should not control price.

The following healthcare services should not enter the market. Market rules should not be used and the government should support these kinds of services (Zhu, 2005):

(1) Healthcare services that aim to prevent diseases.
(2) Basic medical service and primary healthcare determined by the government.
(3) Basic efforts to improve public health, such as the improvement of tap water, and the improvement of facilities for preventing epidemic diseases, etc.
(4) Medical services in the countryside, especially in impoverished areas. It is inappropriate for some provinces and city governments to sell public health centers to solve under-funding problems.
(5) Healthcare services for disabled people or people wounded because of official business.

Of course, defining the boundary between basic medical service and special medical service is difficult. Currently, many problems stem from the fact that there is no effort to distinguish between basic medical services and special medical services. For example, procedures involving surgery are used instead of non-surgical procedures; high-quality antibiotics are used rather than common antibiotics. This is one of the main methods used by hospitals to make a profit. One way to solve the problems induced by the introduction of market mechanisms into the healthcare system is to define what kind of services can be used to make a profit. The initial idea is that market rules will only be applied to a portion of hospital services.

5 Other Recommendations

In recent years, all original state-owned hospitals were defined as non-profit hospitals; very few private clinics were defined as a for-profit hospital. Thus, over 98% hospitals are non-profit hospitals and only 2–3% are for-profit hospitals. This division has resulted in terrible consequences. Small for-profit hospitals cannot compete with non-profit, state-owned hospitals and are eliminated from the market very quickly.

This division provides non-profit hospitals with a big protective umbrella. They still get funding from government, although this is just a small amount. However, they are able to use their formidable superiority to maintain a monopoly in healthcare. They charge high prices, practice deceit, and they cause private hospitals to fail. They use their non-profit status as a protective umbrella to ask for more money from government and to deceive people. This inappropriate division of profit and non-profit hospitals should be corrected immediately in order to establish a normal healthcare market. The majority of state-owned hospitals (60% of the total number of beds) should be defined as for-profit hospitals. The ownership of property rights should be reorganized. If there is no diffusion of property rights, the medical market becomes distorted. A diffusion of property rights will also help these hospitals to enter the market and be managed according to market rules.

The government should increase its funding to non-profit hospitals in order to pay staff, monitor the price of medical services, and compensate the patients for losses possibly brought about by market competition in the medical service. People should be allowed to directly invest in the hospital. Foreign capital should also be allowed to enter the healthcare system.

It should be noted that the current healthcare service market is incomplete, mainly because only the profit mechanism has been introduced. The current healthcare system in our country is mostly a state-owned system; there is no competition in the healthcare system. It is a monopoly; supply and demand does not decide the service price. The current medical market is not a standard market; it is a distorted market, which provides big hospitals with a chance to make huge profits. They are justified in pursuing profits, because the government allows them to use market mechanisms and they are independently managed. However, it is not justifiable for them to not have to pay taxes to the government. Paying taxes is a basic duty for any enterprise. Progressive tax rates have been implemented in most capitalist nations, which is a method of suppressing huge profit taking. Further, these non-profit hospitals still get financial funding from the government and do not have any competitors so that they cannot be forced out from the market. Further, they can freely use every method to increase the hospital's income. This is the precise reason medical expenditures are rising rapidly in our country.

The solution for these problems is to establish a standard medical market with controls and limits. This involves first setting up a profit limit. Hospitals can make a profit but after acquiring a certain amount, the rest must go to the government (The national health department has already implemented such a regulation, but this is not being carried out on a regular basis). The second step is to set a limit on how many beds can be housed in large-scale hospitals to prevent a large number of patients from coming in, and to end the monopoly. The third step is to create a competitive environment to suppress monopoly, rising prices and huge profits. The fourth step is to establish different kinds of hospital ownership systems.

The two-level calculation system in the hospitals should also be canceled. This calculation system requires that each department in a hospital deliver certain amount of money to the hospital administration and anything that exceeds this amount is taken as profit. This system has resulted in excessive medical treatment. This management system is geared toward earning a profit and the hospital becomes like a commercial enterprise. We should explore applying a unification standard to the whole hospital in order to evaluate medical quality, expenses and service attitude.

Also as we have noted earlier, the basic goal of healthcare service is to improve people's health. Healthcare is a basic human right and providing this service for people is the duty of the government. Healthcare should be allocated to as many people as possible. The medical department fails to fulfill its duty if it cannot provide healthcare for the majority of people. To give efficiency and profit priority in the healthcare system is to misunderstand the nature of healthcare. This must be corrected. For this reason, we have to argue that fairness is as important as efficiency and earning a profit in the healthcare system. When the two are opposed to each other, fairness takes priority. This means that hospitals cannot refuse to save a patient's life and throw a patient out of a hospital just because he cannot pay for treatment.

Moreover, a hospital has to consider a patient's ability to pay when deciding whether new techniques and equipment should be used. For example, if a glass-infusing bottle costing 3 Yuan can be used, a plastic infusing bottle costing 11 Yuan should not be used. If there is not much of a qualitative difference between using expensive advanced technology versus using reasonably priced, normal technology, then the normal technology should be used first. Patients should also be allowed to choose what treatments they want. We should eventually formulate standard prices for treatment in order to evaluate whether the hospital is fair. Hospitals that treat many patients at a low cost should be rewarded, and those who treat fewer patients at a higher cost should be punished.

About 10% of hospital profits (including those from non-profit hospitals) should be used to open cheap hospital wards or wards for common people hospitals and they should also be used to aid patients who are incapable of paying their medical bills. A government spending plan should also include some money for hospitals to pay for those kinds of patients.

We should also develop community hospitals; patients with common diseases will be treated in the community hospital. Outpatients should be limited to big hospitals. This measure will stop big hospitals from competing with community hospitals for patients. Currently, patients with common diseases are sent to big hospitals, which results in high medical expenditures.

Regulating the medicine market is also a very important step in establishing a standard medical market. The pharmaceutical market and the medical market should be separately managed. We should follow the international conventions. The mixing up of these two markets cause medical expenditures to surge upward and leads to corruption. The original regulations concerning the separation of the pharmaceutical market and medical services is not practical and should be canceled. We should prohibit the link between the business of promoting drug sales and the prescriptions given by doctors. We should be firmly against doctors receiving sales commission from such procedures. There are no standards in the current pharmaceutical market in our country regarding drug development, production, sales and so on. Different authorities should join together to set up standard in order to stop the corruption.

Finally, the government should increase its investment in the healthcare system in order to strengthen the supervision and management of the healthcare market. It is impossible to establish and introduce market mechanisms into the healthcare system without strong supervision and management from government. Some experts thought the government should stay away from the medical market as far as possible, which is not right. They do not understand the nature of healthcare.

The government is responsible for the following: creating laws and regulations that determine how the medical market should operate, establishing a normal healthcare service market, and preventing people from being deprived of basic healthcare rights. The government should increase its funding for healthcare services like preventative treatment. This is an important step for establishing a moral healthcare system. The government must also increase its funding for non-profit hospitals. If the government does not increase their funding, these hospitals will have to get money from the market, and it will be very difficult to establish an ethical healthcare market.

The government must also increase its funding for the countryside. It is very difficult for the medical services in the countryside to get support from the market. They mainly depend on the government. Government must increase funding for preventative medicine. China is one of the few nations that does not provide much funding for its healthcare system. The current situation should be changed as soon as possible.

6 Trust and Responsibility Are the Foundation of the Doctor–Patient Relationship

In a market economy environment, what is the foundation of the doctor–patient relationship? In addition, how should such a relationship be established? First, trust and responsibility constitute the traditional foundation of the doctor–patient relationship. This is evident when we examine the nature of healthcare. The nature of the medical profession is to cure disease and the healthcare provider must take responsibility for his patient's life. The patient follows the instructions of his doctor. Also in order to get treatment, a patient must sometimes disclose private information to doctors. Therefore, the doctor must gain the trust of his patients. He cannot deceive patients just because his patients lack medical knowledge (Zhu, 1999; Li, 2005, pp. 25–27).

While introducing certain market mechanisms into healthcare complicates the doctor–patient relationship, it does not change the nature of this relationship. Introducing market mechanisms into healthcare does not lessen the importance of the trust that must exist between doctors and patients. It is a misunderstanding to think that introducing certain market mechanisms into healthcare means that the doctor–patient relationship should resemble a business relationship.

Further, although treating illnesses is a service, it is not a service that requires an equal exchange of value. In many situations, doctors provide more than what they are compensated. A doctor often sacrifices his or her own interests to maintain patients' health. Doctors provide what their patients need and not what their patients can pay. Consequently, the government pays for the majority of expenses for those patients who qualify for free medical treatment. Certain impoverished patients get the financial support from both the government and the hospital.

A contractual relationship also exists between the doctor and his patient, but such a relationship is only for preventing disputes. Overemphasizing the contractual and legal relationship only worsens the doctor–patient relationship. Some patients think that because they pay for a doctor's service, they will not be deceived and if they are deceived, then they will try to find any reason to sue their doctors. And some doctors also believe that making money is their goal.

The doctor–patient relationship also deteriorates when patients have impractical requests or when doctors provide nonessential services or fail to provide enough services in order to seek a profit. To resolve conflicts in the current doctor–patient relationship, honesty and trust should be strongly advocated. Lawsuits should only be used in special cases. Even if a problem has to be resolved using legal procedures, trust should be used during the reconciliation process. Massive medical lawsuits can only intensify the conflict.

Consequently, commercial procedures should be completely brandished from medical services. Those include coercing the patient to consent to unessential medical treatments and inspection, propagandizing immature technology, charging the patients unnecessarily, and so forth. Patients must begin to trust doctors and hospitals. They should stop looking for problems so that they can sue.

Also, corruption must be eliminated from all medical services. Doctors must stop accepting red packages, taking sales commissions, and transferring patients to their own clinics. Such behavior seriously hurts the social prestige of the medical profession.

Finally, both doctors and patients should guide their actions according to principle, "If you do not want to be treated a certain way, do not treat others that way." Doctors should show concern for their patients and patients should respect their doctors. Traditional Chinese morals should be widely advocated.

7 To Use Confucius' Beneficence Moral Tradition to Revise the Malady of the Healthcare Market

Presently, the market economy is creating many problems for the healthcare system. How should we deal with the situation? First, we should explore market orders according to healthcare service and set up scientific norms. Second, we need to seek moral guidance (Liang et al., 2005, pp. 1–3).

For moral guidance, we may turn to the moral tradition of Confucianism (kindheartedness) to deal with the problems associated with health care. Specifically, we can turn to the notion of kindheartedness. Confucianism claims that one should always run a country with thoughts of kindheartedness. What are thoughts of kindheartedness? Zigong, one of Confucius' students asked Confucius, "Is it humane to do good things for the masses?" Confucius agreed and said that the meaning of humanity is to benefit both oneself and others. Yanyuan, another of Confucius' students asked the same question. Confucius answered that it is important to restrain selfish desire, and to make one's words and deeds in accordance with etiquette. That is kindheartedness. The famous literati of Tang Dynasty Hanyu summarized the kindheartedness theory of Confucius as follows: universal love is "Ren." Proper realization of "Ren" is "Yi". Going along with kindheartedness is "Dao". To accomplish this and gain trust without the external world is virtue. This view of Confucius provides a solid moral basis for ancient TCM. The famous practitioners of Chinese medicine advocated that medicine is a theory of humanity, the aim of medicine is to cure disease and to save the life of the patient. Today we claim that the aim of medicine is to care for patients and to respect their rights. It is different from the humanitarian theory of Confucius and the moral tradition of TCM. However, it is very important for healthcare to put the patient's interests first. Frankly, if kindheartedness is emphasized more, many problems would be solved. The view that "saving the life of patient is the task of the doctor" may correct the misunderstanding concerning healthcare that arises from market mechanisms. The purpose of introducing some market mechanisms into healthcare is to improve management, not marketization. It does not change hospitals into enterprises nor does it change the aim and purpose of medicine.

We should deal with the relationship of righteousness and benefit by first developing the moral tradition. The problem facing the medical market is the relationship of righteousness and benefit and how to deal with them. When their interests conflict, which takes precedence? Righteousness or benefit? This is a realistic problem. Should benefit take precedence? Doctors and directors of the hospital cannot do that. Of course, we cannot ignore benefits and we should try to strive for a balance of both. When both conflict, we can only reserve "bear's paw and rid of fish," like Mencius said.

We should develop the tradition of universal love. We should treat patients with a kind heart. A market economy thinks that money is what is most important; its face is cool and cruel. Karl Marx said: "a history of Capitalism is a history of fire and blood." He quoted the blood flows from capital and one becomes dirty from head to feet" (Marx, 1976). When we introduce market mechanisms into the health care system, we must be cool and ruthless. We should not cheat patients.

In addition, we should cultivate the thought of caring for the weak. Confucianism stresses the idea that we need "to have equality, no matter what," which reflects the notion that we must care for the weak under the condition of a rural economy. Gong Ting-Xian, a doctor from the Ming Dynasty put forward the suggestion that "curing a patient without discrimination, whether rich or poor is medical justice" (Xia & Hu, 1981, pp. 116–117). The goal of the market is to arouse the enthusiasm of the masses and to develop the economy. However, one disadvantage of the market is that it results in injustice. However, medicine involves the right to life and everyone has the right to health. So therefore, the proper practice of medicine must include justice. At present, the problems of medical justice are conspicuous and China is one of a few countries that do not practice fairness. Precedent measures must be taken to promote medical justice and limit the negative effects of the market economy. Of course, medical justice is not egalitarianism. We do not oppose the idea of the rich enjoying more healthcare services. However, the poor cannot live without rudimental medical services.

When some market mechanisms are introduced into the health care system, we should turn to Chinese moral principles. We should try to make saving patients lives our first goal, limit profits through laws, and insist on justice in the healthcare market. Finally, the doctor–patient relationship should be based on trust and sincerity, and not merely on a business contract. A moral medical market moral may solve many of the problems that we discussed. Any market should be based on moral values, and require moral support and the guarantee of the law. These three elements are interdependent. Morality exists. Values are exchanged and laws are supported. A market without morals is irregular.

References

Annals of China's health. (1990). Beijing: China People's Health Press.

Annals of China's health. (1991). Beijing: China People's Health Press.

Annals of China's health. (1992). Beijing: China People's Health Press.

Annals of China's health. (1998). Beijing: China People's Health Press.

Annals of China's health. (1999). Beijing: China People's Health Press.

Annals of China's health. (2000). Beijing: China People's Health Press.

Annals of China's health. (2001). Beijing: China People's Health Press.

Cao, H., & Fu, J. (2005, August 4). The twenty years of Chinese health care reform. In *South weekend.*

Da, Q. (1999, November). Thinking about some ethical problems in working with medical disputes. In *Medicine and philosophy, 20*, 12.

Du, W. (2000, June 10). The 19 kinds of willful charges which a patient be fallen. In *South weekend.*

Du, Z. (1991). Health care cannot be market. In *Value and society* (2nd ed.). Beijing: China Social Sciences Publishing House.

Fan, M. (1999, May). Perspective of medical disputes. In *Medicine and philosophy, 20*, 17.

Ge, Y. (2005, August 2). State council's developing research center & WHO: On the comment and the suggestions for the Chinese health care reform. In *The times of science and technology, 12*, 2–5.

Guo, Y., & Du, X. (2002, July). The countermeasure for market mechanism and health resources' distribution. In *Medicine and philosophy, 23*, 47–49.

Han, Y., & Cheng, C. (1996). The ethical thought of misapplication of drugs and the retrogression of the quality of life. In *China medical ethics, 9*, (pp. 24–25).

He, L. (2005). To bombard the health care market [Online]. Available: http://www.sina.com.cn. Accessed June 23, 2005.

Liang, H., Guo, Z., & Li, G. et al. (2005, January). The important category of the modern ethics theory: Honest-Trust. In *Chinese medical ethics, 18*, 1–3.

Li, B. (1993). The harassment of "red packs" and the countermeasure. In *Proceedings of 7th national medical ethics symposium.* Zhang Jia Jie city.

Li, S. (2005, June). The conflict between medical personnel and patients and the disappearance of sincerity. In *Medicine and philosophy* (pp. 25–27).

Lu, Q., & Zhou, S. (1993). Medical market and ethics. In *Proceedings of 7th national medical ethics academic symposium.*

Marx, K. (1976). *Capital* (Vol. 1). Harmondsworth: Penguin.

Qing, B. (2000, August 19). The information Center of Ministry of Health: How much is it to see a doctor? In *Dalian daily*.

Ran, Z. (2005). The unsuccessful medical reform. In *Laowan news weekly*, (issue 25).

The center of Chinese communist party and state council's decision of health service's reform and development (1997). In *Annals of China's health* (1998). Beijing: China People's Health Press.

Wang, M. (1993). Hospital health service can neither be marked, nor can be introduced in market mechanisms. In *Proceedings of 7th national medical ethics academic symposium*.

Xia, X., & Hu, G. (1981). The ethics view of Chinese traditional medicine. In *Proceedings of 1st national medical ethics academic symposium*.

Xinghua News Agency. (2001, November 10). Such willful charges 11 big hospitals. In *Southern weekly*.

Zhao, Y. (2000, September). Counting results analysis of the total expenditure of China's health-care. In *Health economy research*.

Zhu, H. (2005). Need to solve seven problems for the health care reform of our country [Online]. Available: http://www.sino.cn. Accessed June 7, 2005.

Zhu, S. (1999, November). New trends of the medical disputes and the countermeasure. In *Medicine and philosophy*.

Markets, Trust, and the Nurturing of a Culture of Responsibility: Implications for Health Care Policy in China

Frederic J. Fransen

1 The Elements of a Culture of Responsibility

The principle elements of a culture of responsibility are biological families, communities, and market relations governing the interactions of families within communities, and of families and communities with one another in society. Each will be looked at in turn.

There are different ways in which to approach the idea of responsibility. Individual responsibility requires that each individual bear the costs of his own actions. Thus, an individual who takes risks – such as driving at high speeds or buying stock in a company – should bear the costs, as well as receive the benefits of those risks. If the driver has an accident, he should be responsible for any damage he causes, and if he injures himself, he should be required to pay the cost of his medical care. Conversely, should an investor's shares in a company return big gains, he should receive those gains, since he bore the risk of loss of his own money.

To most people, this idea of responsibility as individual, however, seems somehow incomplete. It is easy to imagine such a man living alone on an island. Without parents to care for, children to raise, or neighbors to protect, he would bear responsibility for all his actions, but this can only be a limited kind of responsibility, abstracted from the real world in which we live.

A fuller definition of responsibility looks at people as they normally find themselves living together in a group. In this setting, responsibility must in part mean a group of people agreeing to share risks among themselves. That is, they share responsibility. Although there is much to be said for the notion of individual responsibility, since this paper is concerned with policy, it is more appropriate to focus on this latter kind of responsibility within a group. A crucial question for health care and other policy is determining the basic unit of analysis for such groups.

Whereas it is difficult to imagine responsibility in the case of a man alone on an island, it is possible to imagine a responsible family, exhibiting bioethical and moral responsibility, living in isolation on an island. In such a case parents would have

F.J. Fransen, Ph.D.
Liberty Fund, Inc., Indianapolis, IN USA
e-mail: ffransen@libertyfund.org

J. Tao (ed.), *China: Bioethics, Trust, and the Challenge of the Market*,

© Springer Science+Business Media B.V. 2008

responsibilities to create, nurture, and educate their children, and children would later have responsibilities to care for their elderly parents. Moral decisions on how to allocate scarce resources must be made, including their division among unequal children and relatives, and decisions on the appropriate care for sick or injured family members, including the dying. In addition, education for responsibility would be a key moral obligation of parents, particularly so as to inculcate a proper respect for elders as a key to responsible care for the aged.

It is not surprising, then, that in the West, going back at least as far as Aristotle, it has been argued that the primary unit for social analysis is the family. Aristotle writes that the basic unit is the male and female couple, who cannot exist apart from one another (*Politics*, 1252a28–1252b20, Trans. Rackham). In Greek, the word from which the English "economics" is derived is aeconomia, which means "things of the household." Economics as understood in the West, therefore, is at its origin concerned with the material well-being of families. Thus, it is perfectly reasonable to posit the family as the foundational unit of analysis in a culture of responsibility for economic, social, and moral decision-making. The same is true in Confucian tradition.

When we move from mere survival to the question of flourishing, however, it is clear that even families cannot be autarkic, but must interact with others (Aristotle, *Politics*, 1252b20–28, trans. Rackham). Economically, trade among families makes possible a division of labor that allows for massive gains in wealth through increased productivity as well as specialization according to differentiated talents, interests, and skills (Smith, 1981 [1776], pp. 13–24). Such wealth is certainly an important measure of flourishing.

With regard to moral and bioethical questions, communities are necessary to locate and identify appropriate spouses for a family's children outside their immediate biological families. Because children are especially adept at teaching and learning from one another, living within a moral community allows children to be educated in such a way that they learn the values shared by a group of families, either directly through schooling, or perhaps even more importantly in other kinds of social interactions with the children of other adults in the community. This requires a collection of families sharing values and living in close proximity, either physically or through a chain of reliable intermediaries.[1] By extension, therefore, economic, social, and moral life most flourishes in moral communities which may have recognizable physical, geographical boundaries, or be virtual, such as among the Diasporas of many peoples, including the Chinese.

Whereas it is possible for such communities to exist and function as unified economic and moral units, there have been few recent examples of their success over even a single generation, much less across several generations.[2] The market provides an efficient and peaceful mechanism for mediating the interactions among families and communities. Such interaction best occurs in voluntary civil society through market exchange.

Critics of markets often misunderstand them as places in which producers of goods, services, and capital meet with consumers to extort as much profit out of them as possible. According to this understanding, the interests of consumers could better be realized if a central authority took over the productive functions of society – including the production of health care – and either distributed its goods according to their conception of the needs of consumers or regulated their production and distribution according to some optimal formula arrived at by such authorities through central planning.

In recent years, Chinese authorities have realized the weaknesses of the system of central planning that had characterized Chinese economic organization since the introduction of communism, and have made great strides in moving the country forward through the introduction of markets and market-based approaches to economic issues, including the provision of health care. This has not happened without some problems, however.

Although as yet market-based health care reforms have only been partial, in the course of the reforms, observers have already uncovered unpleasant elements within China's health care system, leading to calls for increased market regulation to prevent unethical practices. Some examples include the use of "red packets" – bribes from patients to doctors in return for special services; over-prescription or substitution of more expensive for less expensive medicines; misallocation of resources from socially more important – but less remunerative – to more remunerative uses, and doctors' misdirection of patients from hospitals to private clinics where they have a financial interest.

Critics of markets often lump such ethical and social problems together within the idea of so-called market failure. Such discussions often include notions of "unfair" profit, and calls for caps on "excessive" profit, as well as other government regulation as ways to "correct" for such so-called failures.

Before continuing an account of the role of markets, therefore, I would like to digress a bit and examine more closely this question of "market failure" in the provision of Chinese health care services.

First, it is important to distinguish two very different phenomena in the list of criticisms above. One set of concerns relate to the problem of fraud in doctor–patient relationships, that is, doctors who prescribe medicines, treatments, and facilities which are objectively not appropriate for the illness and patient concerned. This is clearly a great problem not only in doctor–patient situations, but one which characterizes all human relationships. Moreover, it is not a problem unique to China. I will return to this issue later in the paper, when I discuss the problem of trust, and how it should be enforced.

For the purposes of the current discussion of the market and its role, however, a more fundamental criticism concerns the non-fraudulent aspects of market-based health care, namely bribery for services with "red packets" and doctors' pursuit of "excessive profits." I describe these issues as separate from fraud because, although there may be cases in which, for instance, a patience who gives a doctor a "red packet" nevertheless receives sub-optimal care from the doctor, the more theoretically challenging case is one in which the patient offers a "red packet," and actually gets what he believes he is buying in terms of better care. Clearly even this is sometimes deemed inappropriate, and used as a basis for criticism of the market and market reforms.

In order to discuss this issue in terms of the theory of markets, it is crucial to have a clearer understanding of the nature of profit and its role in a properly functioning market economy. Early economic theory, including that of Adam Smith and Karl Marx, looked at economic activity in terms of two inputs: labor and capital. The owner of capital employed the labor of others in order to produce a good or service to sell in the marketplace. The "profit" of the capitalist was the difference between his total costs and the total revenue generated by the sale. Under this understanding, his profit could be excessive if the return on his investment yielded an amount above some determined level.

In order to increase his income, a capitalist had two options: decrease wages or increase prices. To the extent that his ability to do so arose from the weakened circumstances of his employees or his customers, he was taking advantage of them in the pursuit of his own gain. This action may be captured by the Chinese notion of Lì, defined as "profit, gain, advantage." Pursuing this kind of profit raises legitimate ethical concerns not only within Confucian ethics, but also, for example, for Christians, in which concern for others is also a guiding principle of right conduct. If profit were simply gain at the expense of others, it would rightly deserve to be condemned. This in not the whole story, however.

Whereas such a definition of profit has some plausibility in a static world of perfect information, in the real world in which we live it leaves out something vitally important, namely, the role of entrepreneurship in the functioning of an ever-changing economy. Writing in 1911, Joseph Schumpeter described the role of "entrepreneurial profit" in economic development (1934, pp. 128–156). According to Schumpeter, normal economic activity takes place within a circular flow, in which there is no profit. That is, at equilibrium the price of a good includes: the raw materials of production, labor – including the market wages of the businessman for services he might have hired others to do, appropriate (as determined by prevailing market rates) rent, and, finally, interest on capital, whether the entrepreneur uses his own capital or borrows it from others. In an open and competitive market under normal conditions, therefore, many goods are sold at a price that simply captures these things, and leave no "profit" beyond costs of production. Outside times of shortage, commodities such as rice would fit such a description of economic activity as a circular flow, because producers will compete away any additional profit by lowering their prices, and the market price stays very close to the total costs of production.

Economic life, however, is far from static, and the circular flow fails to capture the dynamic side of economic activity, which is crucial for any economy in development, including already highly developed ones. This is always true, but it is particularly so during times of rapid change, such as is the case within Chinese health care today as China introduces more and more market reform. When there are rapid changes in conditions, a great deal of opportunity is opened up for a much more socially productive kind of activity, that of the entrepreneur. Incentives to entrepreneurs come in the form of "entrepreneurial profit." This kind of profit, moreover, should be seen as something desirable within a Confucian understanding, because it is not profit in the sense of taking advantage, but rather is the proper reward provided by the market for activity which is more generally beneficial to mankind.

Let us imagine, for instance, that a physician-entrepreneur has a great many patients with arthritis. He has to choose how to spend his time, and in seeing the extent of that need among his patients, he decides to reallocate his activity away from other tasks toward the development of a new treatment. After considerable effort, he discovers a therapy which is more effective than that currently in use, and begins offering it to his patients. Since the therapy is new, he can set the price where the market will bear it, according to the principles of supply and demand, but as the fame of the new therapy spreads, he has more patients than he can see, and adjusts the price accordingly.

The price for this entrepreneurial product, however, is different from the circular flow price of rice. In this case, in a free market, the price includes raw materials, labor, and interest on capital, but it also includes something more. This "something more" is the "entrepreneurial profit," that arises from the discovery of the therapy. It is important to remember that, in a free market, time and competition will drive away this entrepreneurial profit, so that it is, at best, fleeting. It functions similarly to a temporary monopoly, such as is granted by copyright or patent protection for a limited period of time. For this reason the life of the entrepreneur is precarious. He needs to cover his risk within the short time it will take others to recognize his innovation and copy it, driving away his entrepreneurial profit. Another way of seeing this kind of profit would be to recognize that such "excessive" profit over costs is the reward for innovation. An entrepreneur who becomes wealthy by generating such socially useful innovations is surely engaged in keeping with Yì – right conduct – rather than Lì – advantage. The ethical issue is not that he is being paid well, but that he is paid for socially useful innovation, rather than corrupt activity.[3] We can assume that it is generally socially useful, because he is able to convince consumers to change their customary habits to buy his product, and overcoming the general human resistance to change places a high requirement on him and his innovation.

Finally – to end this digression – it is important to remember that what drives away entrepreneurial profit is transparency and competition in a free market. The existence of "red packets" offered by patients for legitimate services illustrates this. They can only exist where transparency and competition are somehow hindered, probably through misguided government regulation, because otherwise the physician would simply include the amount in his normal fee schedule.[4] Some possible explanations for the presence of "red packets" would include: anti-competitive rules prevent the entry into the market of more physicians offering comparable services; pricing regulations prevent the physician from charging the market price for the service. He is then forced to choose between not offering the service, or including a "red packet" in the price; other barriers prevent the patient from locating an alternative physician, such as prohibitions on advertising one's services; rules governing third-party payers, whether the government or insurance companies, prevent the patient from contracting with the physician to provide the service at the market price. For instance, the government might restrict certain patient to using physicians in their village or town, even if the service is not available there, and restrict physicians from seeing patients from other areas.

Each of these examples of the explanation for the existence of "red packets" is not an example of market failure, but rather of a failure to allow markets to do what they do best – to allocate scarce resources in a complicated world.

In his seminal essay "The Use of Knowledge in Society," Friedrich Hayek (1948 [1945], pp. 77–91) has shown that government direction of economic activity – whether in the form of actual planned economies or through regulations that interfere with the free functioning of the market – is based upon a fundamentally flawed understanding of the basic problem of economics and the actual role played by markets. According to Hayek, the basic problem of economic organization is how rapidly to transmit complex information about changes in conditions affecting supply and demand to those who can use it to adjust their production or consumption. The problem planners and regulators face is that useful economic knowledge cannot be captured in the aggregate data available to them, but rather is only known – and can only be known – by widely dispersed economic agents, in effect, by each producer and consumer separately. Since, as was noted above, the fundamental economic unit is the family, this means that only families have enough economic information to arrive at appropriate economic decisions, including decisions about health care.

How do they communicate this information? The answer, Hayek argues, is by means of prices. The price mechanism, according to Hayek, is really an ingenious device, discovered accidentally by man, to transmit vast amounts of information about economic conditions to those who can make use of it, without requiring any specialized knowledge of the specific conditions causing changes in supply and demand to be known by more than a few people, or perhaps by any one person at all. As prices change, people alter their purchasing habits to adjust in the most appropriate way to changes in underlying economic conditions. If a price goes up, it tells them to look for substitutes for the good in question. If prices go down, they consider using more of the less expensive goods as a substitute for others whose prices have remained the same. All each buyer needs to know is what, for him and his family, are the appropriate substitute goods, and he can make the best possible decisions, given his circumstances. Most importantly, accepting or refusing to buy a good at a given price transmits crucial information about scarcity and demand in a better way, Hayek argues, than any other system discovered by man.

As one example, China has an extremely unequal distribution of physicians and medical resources across the country. As a result, the price charged for the same service can vary widely from place to place, along with its availability. This presents a problem to the country, but also an entrepreneurial opportunity. One might imagine a company providing transportation services to bring doctors to needy areas, with the patients offering a premium to cover the costs of doing so. In some instances, one might also imagine that same company transporting patients to where the doctors are located. Price differentials between locations provide opportunities to pay innovators for the time, effort, and risk involved in devising means to alleviate this problem. This might be as simple as providing a directory of underutilized doctors, or a table of comparative prices for services in different areas, as a way of helping medical producers and consumers find one another. Moreover, the ability of such a health-care entrepreneur to adjust to varied and changing needs will almost certainly exceed that of a regulator, because his livelihood will depend upon making good decisions, and if he does not, he will be forced out of business, leaving an opening for someone else with better information to replace him.

Now, if prices are really bits of information about relative scarcity, transmitted along the chain from producers to suppliers, what role do markets play? First, markets are places – physical or virtual – where people come together to engage in exchange based upon their desires, given a set of relative prices. This is a very delicate process, because those desires are often affected by the prices themselves, so markets provide a very intricate feedback mechanism to help people maximize their ability to fulfill their (varied) desires. In order for the price mechanism to convey accurate information, these prices – and the exchanges that take place based upon them – need to be arrived at voluntarily. In any real market, exchange can and will only take place if each party believes that the object he receives is of more value to him than the one which he is offering in trade. Thus, markets are places in which people come together to transmit information by trading things they consider of less value for those they consider to be of more value. At the end of every voluntary exchange, although nothing new is produced, both parties have increased their wealth, as they understand it. For families to flourish, they must be able to learn about scarcity so as to adjust their own consumption, as well as to be able to exchange goods of less value for those of more value. For this reason, markets are central to any family or community desiring to flourish. Markets in health care are no exception to this general rule.

In addition to families, communities, and markets, the final element necessary to build a culture of responsibility is a reliable system of trust. This might be described as the rule of law, and it has two components.

First, whenever one agrees to engage in an exchange in the marketplace, he must trust that others with whom he is trading will reliably uphold their end of the agreement. This might be as simple as knowing that when I hand you money to buy a piece of fruit, you will, indeed, give me the fruit. Or it might involve very complicated loans and promises of paying rent over many years so that I can construct a commercial building and pay a long chain of builders and suppliers. In either case, to preserve order, it is crucial for a third party to act as a guarantor so that both of us know if you don't give me the fruit, I don't have to use force to take it from you, but can appeal to that third party to do so on my behalf. Although one might imagine situations in which such agreements can be enforced without a single central authority, in practice this is the responsibility of the state.

The second element of trust concerns the state itself. In order to calculate risk and engage in long-term planning – including intergenerational planning – it is important to be able to trust the state not only to enforce contracts among families and communities, but also to protect the property of those families and communities from one another, as well as from the state itself. That is, for families and communities to flourish, the state must not only prevent theft among families, but must also restrain itself from taking the property of those families, beyond reasonable[5] taxation and fees.

This principle of restraint by the government is well-illustrated in the writings of Mencius[6] (1970, p. 99): "Benevolent government must begin with land demarcation. When boundaries are not properly drawn, the division of land according to the well-field system and the yield of grain used for paying officials cannot be equitable. For this reason, despotic rulers and corrupt officials always neglect the boundaries."

In other words, codifying and enforcing property rights is the first principle of good government. Moreover, Mencius also used this occasion to establish the proper rate of taxes for a benevolent government to collect. According to the well-field system, each farmer's land should be evenly divided into nine pieces, with the product of the center piece worked for the government and the rest being retained for the use of the family. Today, this would convert into a flat tax of 11%. This should be looked upon as an upper limit on legitimate taxation, with all government activity based upon compulsory taxation – whether for public security or transfers to the needy and infirm – confined to this level.

For good government these are not only necessary conditions, they are also sufficient ones, provided that the government uses those taxes it collects prudently. When it does not – either through excess collection or improper allocation of those taxes – it does so at the cost of a family-centered culture of responsibility.

Finally, to apply the issue of trust directly to the question of health and health care policy, it is interesting to note the prominent place this plays in traditional Chinese ethics. In his paper, Li Benfu provides important insights into the status of trust in the doctor–patient relationship, while lamenting the apparent decline in that trust in recent years. Although it is tempting to suggest that market reform has played a role in the decline of trust as more and more patients have begun to question the motives of their physicians, one should be cautious about this interpretation.

In order to examine this issue, one can return to the question of "red packets" and look at the question first raised above. Suppose a patient gives a "red packet" to a physician, but instead of receiving the promised better care in return, he receives sub-optimal care. For our purposes here, the main concern is the fraud which has been perpetrated, not the bribe. Under such circumstances, it is unlikely that the patient will appeal to the government to enforce the promise, because to do so would require explain the initial, presumably illegal, use of a "red packet." As a result, the fraud goes unnoticed, and therefore unpunished, not only by the state, but also by other consumers.

Compare with this the reaction of the market to the production of faulty goods. As people learn that the product they are receiving is not worth the price, they begin to buy less of that product, whether it is a medicine or the latest consumer electronics device. The producer can respond by lowering the price, but that itself sends a signal to other consumers than this product is less valuable than comparable ones. In a free market, it is very difficult to engage in fraud for long, because every consumer acts as an enforcer, and the transparency that real prices affords sends them better signals about relative value. In a free market, someone asking for an outside payment is prima facie evidence that one should be suspicious. In a non-market economy it is impossible to know, because there are no real prices. Free markets, therefore, not only help to build trust by providing transparency, they also eliminate the incentives to engage in distrustful activity which government regulation provides. It is almost certain, therefore, that the use of "red packets" predates market reforms and is a remnant of earlier practices, rather than caused by the market.

2 Alternative Views of a Culture of Responsibility Centered on the Family and Community: The Amish

Many philosophers would prefer that the state, instead of families, play a much larger role than that described above and are not hesitant to express their willingness to interfere with the responsibility of families and communities to make decisions. They argue that their preference for centralized, uniform, democratic schemes for education, health care, and care for the elderly justify denying to families and communities decision-making authority in these areas. In order to explore just how unfriendly to families and communities such political theory can be, I will now explore the intolerance of a number of philosophers, followers of John Rawls, to one particular community, the Amish of North America.

The choice of the Amish is designed to be illustrative, but it is not arbitrary. The Amish's unapologetic defense of their right as families and communities to educate their children, to finance and provide health care for their members and their families, and to care for their elderly – the prime elements of any health care policy – make them exemplars for those seeking to create a society based around families living out a culture of responsibility. Moreover, their stubbornness in the face of outside attacks provide considerable evidence of the threat that responsible families and communities pose to some worldviews, and in particular to Rawlsian ones.

The Amish trace their origins to a group of Swiss men and women who, in 1525, declared that a moral and religious community should be voluntary, and that entry into such a community should not follow automatically upon one's birth, but rather should be entered into only by freely-choosing adults. The generic name for this group is "Anabaptist." Anabaptist communities include not only the Amish but also Mennonites, Brethren, and Hutterites. There are about 180,000 Amish living in the United States and Canada, mostly in small, farming communities. Although they are often thought of as inward-looking, with regard to bioethical issues, they are generous to outsiders. For instance, they are avid organ donors, and give blood at levels considerably above that of the general population. In addition, as a population that had only about 5,000 members in 1900 and that is effectively committed to marriage within the community, they have a remarkably homogenous gene pool, making them useful subjects for studies on genetic transmission of disease; they are also generous in donating tissue and blood samples for such studies.

Amish life is built around large, biological families. These families are organized in districts, averaging 35 families each. A leader chosen by lot oversees every two districts. The Amish exhibit a great deal of responsibility over issues of health care for their community (Huntington, 1993, pp. 163–190). Most births occur at home or in Amish birthing centers, with many deliveries conducted by unlicensed midwives. The Amish provide their children with education through the eighth grade, usually in one-room Amish schools (Meyers, 1993, pp. 87–108). They avoid buying health insurance, but rather self-insure when they need to use outside medical facilities or see doctors. With regard to various health care protocols, they generally accept the principles of modern medicine,[7] but are reluctant to accept radical measures to prolong life, preferring to let nature run its course and to die at home in the care of their family. Mentally ill members are integrated into the work of the community if possible, and often cared for at home, although the Amish have also begun to establish their own facilities to care for the severely mentally ill. In order to care for the elderly, it is customary for a special house to be built on the property of one of the children, usually the oldest son, where the parents live and are cared for until they die.

The Amish cultivate such self-sufficiency out of an ethic of voluntary separation from society at large. They believe that they can live a better life apart, and in return for not bothering others, they insist upon not being bothered themselves. Their relationship with society is unidirectional. That is, they are generous in helping strangers, but are reluctant to accept outside help, particularly from any government, because they see such help as interfering with their family-centered and community-based culture of mutual responsibility.[8] This refusal has brought them into frequent conflict with the U.S. government. Here are just a few of the issues with consequences for health care policy upon which they have taken principled stands in order to preserve the integrity of their communities:

Social Security: Social Security is the American government program of support for the elderly, along with the unemployed, disabled, and a few other categories. The program is paid for with taxes specially collected for it, adding up to about 15% of income. Although the Amish willingly pay other taxes on property, sales, and income, Social Security is particularly troublesome for them because they believe that families – and when families are unable, the district or even the Amish community as a whole – should be responsible for caring for the elderly, sick, and disabled among them. After a long fight, in 1965 they were granted exemption from paying Social Security taxes, and in 1978 this was extended to Amish who work as employees.

Insurance: By extension, the Amish are also reluctant to participate in insurance programs of any kind, including health insurance, preferring instead to rely on one another in times of need. Instead of commercial insurance, as a matter of moral principle, the Amish help each other with donations when a particular family suffers an unbearable hardship, whether it is with regard to health, the loss of property due to fire, or some other event. Their mutual aid is not only monetary, but also takes the form of helping to rebuild barns and houses destroyed by fire or storm, volunteering time to care for the sick or disabled, etc.

Education: Perhaps the most controversial issue with regard to the Amish has been their stance on education. Believing that schooling beyond basic education in reading, writing, and arithmetic is unnecessary and, moreover, threatening to their community, they have insisted that their children generally end their formal education after 8 years of school and instead concentrate on practical education on their farms or places of business. Because many states have laws mandating children attend school until age sixteen or older, this has led to serious disputes with government officials. In 1972, however, in a case known as Wisconsin vs Yoder, the United States Supreme Court sided with the Amish and created a special provision allowing Amish families to withdraw their children from school at age fourteen, after the eighth grade. As we will see below, this ruling has been widely criticized by Rawlsian political theorists, and this issue will serve as an example of why a strongly family-oriented culture is incompatible with Rawlsian theory.

Three additional aspects of the Amish understanding of a culture of responsibility based around the family are worth noting. First, the Amish have an unusual understanding of decision-making structures.[9] Families are patriarchal. Routine community decisions are referred to a leader chosen from among eligible men by lot. Important decisions, such as whether to expel a member for disobedience, are reserved for the near-unanimous consent of all members, with women having an equal voice with men. Outside their communities, however, the Amish generally abstain from any involvement in political activity, whether it be voting, suing in courts, or serving in government jobs, including in the military. Finally, although they take little or no part in the social or political life of wider society, the Amish participate fully in the economic life around them. Each family, which usually consists of several different generations, functions as an economic unit. They sometimes use peculiar production methods and typically work in agriculture, but they have developed niche markets in cabinetry, carpentry, and other skilled crafts. Increasingly, they also work in factories, and sometimes own and operate large businesses.

None of this would be relevant if the Amish were not thriving, or their way of life was not considered desirable to their members. Although few outsiders join the Amish, and despite the fact that they require their children to live outside the moral control of their communities for a period of 2–6 or more years before they are allowed voluntarily to join, today more than 90% of children born of Amish parents do voluntarily choose to join, once they are old enough to make a conscious, free choice and have had enough experience with the outside world for that choice to be informed. By any objective standard, therefore, they provide examples of successful, family-based communities which foster and develop a culture of responsibility.

The ability of the Amish to flourish in the United States has largely rested on a combination of the guarantee of their freedom of religion, and basic protections for economic freedom. In no way has it relied upon democratic principles. Indeed, as mentioned above, although the Amish would be allowed to participate in political decision-making (voting and holding office) in the United States, they do not consider doing so to be necessary to their way of life, and, indeed, they consider such participation to be intrinsically dangerous to the preservation of their communities.[10]

Although it is not the purpose of this paper to develop a robust political theory in which family-based communities such as the Amish might flourish, I would only point to the idea of a framework society as described by Robert Nozick in his famous book, Anarchy, State, and Utopia (1974) for an example of such a theory.[11] Nozick's essay was a direct response to one of the most influential philosophers of the twentieth century, John Rawls. Rawls' early work was intended to design a political and social system based around the notion of equality of opportunity. Recognizing that different individuals have different innate abilities, Rawls tried to develop a system that would guarantee that the places such individuals found in society was dependent entirely upon their ability, rather than the result of unfair advantages or disadvantages due to any quality except merit. Where differences did exist, social institutions ought to be designed so as to mitigate the effects of these differences on social outcomes.

Students of Rawls have extended his arguments in a number of interesting, but ultimately shocking, ways for those who seek to support families. For instance, James Fishkin (1983, pp. 50–67) argues that if one truly desires to prevent a child from receiving unfair advantages based on accident of birth, one must greatly limit the rights of the biological family. This might be done by randomly assigning babies to different parents, or severely limiting the rights of parents to give their child "unfair" advantages, for instance by providing extra help with schoolwork or vacations to culturally and historically important places. In so many words, Fishkin suggests that a Rawlsian understanding of justice demands radical limitations on the responsibility and liberty of families, if not their complete destruction.

Fishkin does not refer specifically to the Amish, but many other authors do. Most of their writings have as a backdrop a rejection of Wisconsin vs Yoder, in which the U.S. Supreme Court declared that the Amish did not need to send their children to school beyond age fourteen. The arguments against the Amish fall into three categories: (1) they actively interfere with the ability of the state to expose all children to alternative ways of life so that they can make autonomous decisions about how to live; (2) they fail to teach children to use "critical reasoning" to evaluate the appropriateness of their family's and community's values; and (3) the Amish hinder their children from learning the skills necessary to participate in the political life of the (democratic) state by refusing to allow them to attend more than 8 years of school.

The first part of this argument focuses on the "right" of children to be exposed to different worldviews so as to be able to make autonomous decisions about which one they prefer. For example, Amy Gutmann (1980, p. 349) argues that the state has a right to compel children to attend certain kinds of schools so that they will be exposed to different values and worldviews: "A child's right to compulsory education is a precondition to becoming a rational human being and a full citizen of a liberal democratic society." As a result, according to Gutmann, Amish children have a "right" to be forced – against their will and that of their parents – to attend certain kinds of schools.

Especially telling for health care policy is Gutmann's list (1980, p. 356) of which rights the state should protect, and which it should deny to children. For instance, the state should protect children's rights to abortion and medical care against their family's wishes, and even their right to leave their families altogether. But the child should not be allowed the right to opt out of Gutmann's educational system. While not stating that it should be rejected, Gutmann (2003, p. 183) implies that Wisconsin vs Yoder was mistaken, and rightly recognizes that her system of democratic control over education could not be sustained if the rights Wisconsin vs Yoder recognized for the Amish were extended to all families.

Rather than making an argument about being exposed to a wide range of choices, Richard Arneson and Ian Shapiro (1996) instead emphasize the requirement that democratic citizens be educated in critical reasoning skills so that they can make reasoned decisions for themselves and within a democratic polity, including especially the decision whether or not to join a group such as the Amish. They argue that the Amish aversion to state education is explicitly designed to deny critical reasoning skills to their children, and that for this reason, the decision in Wisconsin v. Yoder is incompatible with their theory of democratic education.[12]

Areneson and Shapiro's worry about the Amish avoiding training in a certain kind of critical reasoning is only partly out of concern for the freedom of their choice whether to join or not join an Amish community. As they write (Areneson & Shapiro, 1996, p. 404), "autonomy and democracy go together," and critical reasoning is also necessary to "participate effectively in democratic deliberation." Therefore, unless the Amish go to high school, Areneson and Shapiro worry, they won't have sufficient reasoning skills to be competent to vote and hold office. This is an interesting argument, because given the ability of the Amish to engage in other sorts of critical reasoning – from an understanding of the nature of genetically inheritable diseases which encourages them to participate in biomedical studies, to their ability successfully to compete in agricultural production against others using sophisticated farming techniques, it would seem that the Amish exhibit some kind of critical reasoning, if not the kind which appeals to Areneson and Shapiro. Presumably, then, Areneson and Shapiro have a particular kind of critical reasoning in mind, one which only a very particular kind of education can provide. If this is correct, as an alternative to rounding up Amish children and carting them off to high school against their will, one might suggest, for example, that the government establish a "critical reasoning" test which all would-be voters (not just the Amish) must pass in order to vote or hold office. This might, of course, prevent the Amish from voting,[13] but since they generally opt out of democratic decision making and political society anyway, denying them voting rights would not be a severe hardship, nor have any kind of detrimental effect on their communities.

This leads to the question of whether it is possible for Rawlsian liberalism to tolerate a family-centered community such as the Amish at all. The answer is, at best, reluctantly. Authors such as Areneson, Shapiro and Gutmann accept that the stakes are low and the influence of the Amish small enough that it is not worth forcing them to change. The same view is held by advocates of Rawls' later, seemingly more tolerant, theory of "political liberalism," such as Stephen Macedo (1995, pp. 488, 496), who argues that one "cannot be entirely happy about accommodating the Amish," but although they shouldn't be banned, they must "pay a price" for such accommodation. Will Kymlicka (2001, p. 170) takes this one step further, arguing explicitly that Wisconsin vs Yoder was wrongly decided. Kymlicka also states that since the Amish are here and came under certain conditions, they should not be expelled, but he demands that no similar group be allowed to immigrate again without explicitly giving up their rights to family-centered education and related practices.

By now it should be evident that Rawlsian liberalism is at best in great tension, and mostly likely incompatible, with a strong, family-centered culture of responsibility as exemplified by the Amish.[14] For many of the same reasons, this is also true of Juergen Habermas's (1993) notion of "discursive democracy" and any other theory which requires active, uniform participation in political and social life. The reason is that such theories place few or no limits on the ability of political bodies to intrude into community or family life. Nor do they have an easy way of allowing families and communities to make different choices from that of the society as a whole. By not ruling out interference in families, they replace family or community responsibilities with political solutions to problems such as child-rearing, care for the elderly, and health care.[15]

This, finally, takes us back to Hayek's comments on the dispersal of economic knowledge. If the relevant information to make a decision for a family can only be fully understood by that family, then submitting such a decision to political debate and control cannot produce a better solution than if the family were left to decide according to its own procedures. Furthermore, it follows implicitly that if one is no longer allowed to make economic decisions, one cannot be held responsible, either. As a result, denying families economic responsibility – including responsibility for health care decisions and the costs associated with them – makes a culture of responsibility impossible to sustain over the long term.

There are a number of aspects of German culture that, for reasons similar to those described above, work against Germany supporting a family-centered culture of responsibility. I will simply mention two here: German inheritance law makes it difficult – or nearly impossible – for families to make decisions about who should inherit what on any basis but that of equality. This not only undermines the authority of the family, but also reduces incentives to cultivate responsibility. Second, German education law requires what the Rawlsians seek in American education law, namely, it prohibits virtually all alternatives to centrally controlled and politically managed schools. Under such conditions, it is difficult or impossible to raise children in an ethic of responsibility.

3 Freedom for Families and Communities as the Key Element to Fostering a Culture of Responsibility

If China, then, seeks to create an environment that nurtures families and communities in a culture of responsibility, what are the key elements it should promote? First, as the paper makes clear, of central importance is the creation of an institutional framework in which economic decision-making is left to individual families or family groups, because they are best able to make use of the decentralized knowledge necessary to produce a wealthy and flourishing society. For families to be able to make appropriate decisions, they will need a state which protects their property not only from theft and other breaches of contract between citizens, but also offers a stable environment in which the state itself refrains from interfering with the property rights of those citizens, except in predictable, limited, and prudent ways.

To what models, then, might China look in designing particular policies? Given the centrality of economic freedom, a good place to start would be the countries listed at the top of one or the other of the Economic Freedom Indices.[16] These two indices use slightly different methodology and have somewhat different rankings of countries, but generally reach similar conclusions about the economic freedom of various countries. Hong Kong is at the top of both lists. Presumably, the important institutional features of Hong Kong are either well-known or easily studied in China. Hopefully Hong Kong will continue to maintain its ranking in years to come.

The second ranked country Singapore, however, might also offer lessons that China might wish to consider. Singapore is an interesting model because in addition to having the highest degree of economic freedom in the world outside Hong Kong, it also has a policy intentionally designed to foster the preservation of family and community responsibility (Tan, 2004). Taxation is low, allowing families to accumulate wealth, and wide discretion is given to families in the distribution of inheritance. Education is decentralized, and Singapore's various communities are not required to engage in education contrary to their religious and moral beliefs. Furthermore, although there are some government safety nets, by and large the constitutional and legal framework of Singapore encourages communities to engage in mutual aid and support rather than rely upon centralized, government insurance for health, welfare, and other social concerns. Its laws have been successful in encouraging families and communities to develop associations and institutions that are essential to any culture of responsibility. For this reason it is fair to say that, in principle at least, whereas family-centered communities such as the Amish are under attack in the United States and could not live in Germany, they would be at home in the institutional setting offered by Singapore.[17]

4 Health Care Policy for a Culture of Responsibility

Finally, drawing on the arguments put forward above, what are the most important elements specific to health care policy that would be required to foster a culture of responsibility? I offer three:

Bioethical decision-making should be left to appropriate community and/or family decision-making structures, and economic units (families) should bear responsibility for the economic costs of health care. To the extent that this is not possible for particular individual cases, within the 11% limit on legitimate taxation, government should engage in transfers through medical savings accounts or some similar device, rather than insurance or insurance-like schemes, so as to maximize ownership and responsibility on the part of the recipients.

Risk-sharing (such as with insurance) should appropriately rest at the level of voluntary moral communities, in which health-relevant (and other) norms are best determined.

The institutional structure for health care delivery should use the market to provide services, and allow market forces to allocate resources among communities.

5 Conculsion

Appropriate structures for a market-based culture of responsibility for health care delivery exist in some places, but are under attack by Rawlsians and their allies, in the United States, Germany and elsewhere. China has the opportunity to lead the world in the development of policies that would nurture a culture of responsibility in health care, if it is willing to allow families and communities to be the locus of decision-making and financing of health care, and to allow market forces to provide society-level allocation of resources among families and communities.

Notes

[1] Thus it is fully appropriate, and not unusual, for immigrants to look to their home countries to provide guidance and assistance in locating suitable spouses for themselves and their children.

[2] One exception is the Hutterites of North America. A significant element of their success, however, is probably due to the strict limitations they place on size, such that each moral/economic unit consists of no more than about thirty families. Among their wider communities, economic decision-making is not coordinated in any day-to-day way.

[3] Some of this activity, while constructive to consumers, may be harmful to individual competitors. The invention of antibiotics and sterile technique was harmful to the nursing industry, because it greatly reduced the number of patients in hospitals or otherwise requiring care while recovering from infections. Schumpeter referred to this as the "creative destruction" brought about by entrepreneurial activity, and used this to explain the animosity which is often generated toward entrepreneurs. Markets are powerful tools for eliminating less productive producers. This is particularly applicable to the economics of hospitals, which appears to be a central concern in debates about Chinese health care policy. The relevant issue is the competitive status of government vs private, and profit vs non-profit hospitals. There is no reason, a priori, to privilege one or the other legal or management structure. What is important is that they all, regardless of their legal status, have to compete on an even playing field. This means no subsidies for any of them, including the government hospitals, and especially no protection against bankruptcy. The market is at least as "productive" when it is weeding out unsuccessful producers as when it is creating new ones to replace them.

[4] Presumably payments in the form of "red packets" are illegal. Thus, presumably there are incentives such that, all other things being equal, both physician and patient would prefer open payment.

[5] What is reasonable taxation, of course, is subject to dispute. In the West, there is a long tradition which argues that taxation up to a rate of 10% is legitimate, but that anything beyond 10% is unacceptable.

[6] I am especially grateful to Julia Tao for pointing out these very important insights of Mencius. Please see Tao (2006) for a fuller discussion of the ethical implications of the well-field system.

[7] The Amish apply a kind of moral precautionary principle to health care innovation. That is, rather than allowing a new technique or procedure to be used without question, they examine it to see whether it is in keeping with their moral values. If they are persuaded that it is, then they will adopt it. Thus, although they were initially skeptical about the value of many immunizations, they have

been persuaded that it is important for public health to do so, and now generally allow themselves to be vaccinated. It is interesting that in this case it was important to argue that it would be harmful to *others* not to be vaccinated, and it was in keeping with their desire to be generous in their regard for strangers, rather than out of concern for their own safety, that compelled them to accept immunization programs.

8 This unidirectional ethic can be illustrated in looking at the way they discipline their members, a practicing known as "shunning." When a member violates one of the rules of the community, upon a vote of the members, he is "shunned." This means that he is temporarily considered outside the community. During this time, members can offer help and assistance *to* the shunned member, but cannot accept anything – including food, transportation, or marital relations, *from* that member, until he is restored to good standing.

9 One should note that each community is self-governing, so that the rules vary somewhat from one group of Amish to another.

10 Hegel (1991 [1821], p. 295) recognized as much when he said that Anabaptists were members only of civil society, not the state.

11 Another philosopher whose theory is compatible with the Amish is William Galston (1991, 2002).

12 Arneson and Shapiro base their case that the Amish oppose the teaching of critical reasoning to their children on testimony from the case itself, along with a comment in Donald J. Kraybill's description of the Amish, *The Riddle of Amish Culture* (2001) in which Kraybill argues that Amish children are socialized in such a way that when they do decide to join the community, their choice is not meaningfully free. This is a strong criticism, and Kraybill's claim deserves further study. It may be that sociologists and philosophers have different understandings of "free," and one useful place to start would be to explore whether the not infrequent choices of Amish children *not* to join the community are equally unfree, and if so how.

13 Although it might turn out that on any conceivable, value-neutral test, Amish children might score better than average. Thomas Meyers refers to studies that determined that Amish children perform better than non-Amish in standardized tests in spelling, word usage, and arithmetic. (1993, p. 105).

14 Although most of the venom against the Amish focuses on their exemption from schooling, it is fair to presume that the same arguments against the Amish in this regard can be extended to their refusal to participate in Social Security and other national insurance programs.

15 Moreover, in their effort to arrive at agreement through discursive political procedures, Habermas prioritizes thought over action. For a group such as the Amish, however, community life is built around deeds and actions, not talk, and to be forced to engage in debate so as to be able to arrive at a political solution to some problem is itself a threat to the Amish understanding of responsibility.

16 The Fraser Institute in Canada: http://www.freetheworld.com/ and Heritage Foundation in the United States: http://www.heritage.org/research/features/index/

17 Many in the West are critical of Singapore's limitations on political rights. As has been mentioned above, however, whatever value political rights might have for other purposes, for nurturing a culture of responsibility they pale in comparison to economic rights, in which Singapore excels.

References

Arneson, R. J., & Shapiro, I. (1996). Democratic autonomy and religious freedom: A critique of Wisconsin v. Yoder. *Nomos, 38*, 365–411.

Fishkin, J. S. (1983). *Justice, equal opportunity, and the family*. New Haven: Yale.

Galston, W. A. (1991). *Liberal purposes: Goods, virtues, and diversity in the liberal state.* New York: Cambridge University Press.

Galston, W. A. (2002). *Liberal pluralism: The implications of value pluralism for political theory and practice*. New York: Cambridge University Press.

Gutmann, A. (1980). Children, paternalism, and education: A liberal argument. *Philosophy and Public Affairs, 9*, 338–358.

Gutmann, A. (2003). *Identity in democracy*. Princeton, NJ: Princeton University Press.

Habermas, J. (1993). *Justification and application: Remarks on discourse ethics*. New York: Cambridge University Press.
Hayek, F. (1948 [1945]). *Individualism and economic order* (pp. 77–91). Chicago: University of Chicago.
Hegel, G. W. F. (1991 [1821]). *Elements of the philosophy of right*. New York: Cambridge University Press.
Huntington, G. E. (1993). Health care. In D. B. Kraybill (Ed.), *The Amish and the state* (pp. 163–190). Baltimore: Johns Hopkins University Press.
Kraybill, D. B. (2001). *The riddle of Amish culture*. Baltimore: Johns Hopkins University Press.
Kymlicka, W. (2001). *Politics in the Vernacular: Nationalism, multiculturalism and citizenship*. New York: Oxford University Press.
Macedo, S. (1995). Liberal civic education and religious fundamentalism: The case of God v. John Rawls? *Ethics, 105*, 468–496.
Mencius (1970 [ca. 319 B.C.]). *Mencius*. In D.C. Lau (trans.). New York: Penguin.
Meyers, T. J. (1993). Education and schooling. In D. B. Kraybill (Ed.), *The Amish and the state* (pp. 87–108). Baltimore: Johns Hopkins University Press.
Nozick, R. (1974). *Anarchy, state, and Utopia*. New York: Basic Books.
Schumpeter, J. A. (1934 [1911]). *The theory of economic development: An inquiry into profits, capital, credit, interest, and the business cycle*. Cambridge: Harvard University Press.
Smith, A. (1981 [1776]). *An inquiry into the nature and causes of the wealth of nations*. Indianapolis: Liberty Fund.
Tan, K. (2004). The legal and institutional framework and issues of multiculturalism in Singapore. In L. A. Eng (Ed.), *Beyond rituals and riots: Ethnic pluralism and social cohesion in Singapore* (pp. 98–113). Singapore: Eastern Universities Press.
Tao, J. (2006). Confucian foundations of trust and responsibility. In J. Tao (Ed.), *China: Bioethics, trust, and the challenge of the market* (pp. 75–87). Dordrecht: Springer.

Fostering Professional Virtue in the Market: Reflections on the Challenges Facing Chinese Health Care Reform

Jeremy Garrett*

1 Introduction

Free markets are anonymous; they allow individuals with radically different goals, purposes, and understandings of virtue to trade goods and services peacefully and efficiently. Free markets are not only efficient means for allocating goods and services; they also tend to stimulate the production of new goods and services. Markets are the mother of innovation and creation. Although markets possess all these important advantages in general and for health care in particular, they do not of themselves directly support attitudes that lead to attentive care for customers, especially when those customers are patients. Nor do they directly lead to the nurturing of moral integrity. As a consequence, when customers are patients, one may have concerns about the role of the market in the provision of health care, as well as about giving a central place to private health care institutions.

This essay argues that such concerns, although they are sincere and they identify important moral issues, are often misplaced. In fact, on closer examination, the bond between markets and care for customers (in this case patients) turns out to be more significant than might at first blush be anticipated. There are good reasons to hold that, in a health care market with appropriate supporting institutions, these and similar concerns will be met. In particular, where (1) health care consumers have good data regarding quality of care and the integrity of health care professionals and (2) where the rule of law is taken seriously, private health care institutions and providers will nurture, not undermine, the quality of health care. At stake are two central but complex insights regarding human social and economic activity: (1) Mandeville's recognition that "private vices can produce public benefits" and (2) Adam Smith's metaphor of the "invisible hand." The point is that the free and private pursuit of market gain, what Mandeville provocatively refers to as the pursuit of "vice," along with what Smith characterizes as the pursuit of "self-interest," can

J. Garrett
Assistant Professor in the Department of Philosophy, California State University, Sacramento, Sacramento, California
e-mail: garrettj@rice.edu

* Jeremy Garrett is Senior Managing Editor, *The Journal of Medicine and Philosophy*

J. Tao (ed.), *China: Bioethics, Trust, and the Challenge of the Market*,

© Springer Science+Business Media B.V. 2008

often (unintentionally) engender a higher overall quality of health care, professional virtue, and stronger commitments to moral integrity within a large-scale population than comparable public institutions that are, from their very conception or reconstruction, deeply and intentionally structured by "rational" principles of just social organization.[1]

More specifically, this essay argues that this general thesis regarding markets is defensible even when applied to a country as sizable and complex as China, where transitioning to more market-based systems for health care delivery might seem to present particularly daunting challenges. For example, many might understandably worry that installing market reforms will inevitably erode the Confucian values that have long structured Chinese attitudes regarding health care, perhaps replacing them with more Western values like commitments to radical individualism. Or, to address another issue, many no doubt have concerns that markets will foster greater exploitation of the more vulnerable and poorer populations of rural China than will state-run health care bureaucracies. Such worries are serious and not to be dismissed cavalierly. However, it is equally important to note that they do not represent essential properties of markets, in general, or health care markets, in particular. Moreover, not only are such adverse moral outcomes not essential properties of markets, they are not even particularly probable outcomes, so long as there is a strong commitment to the rule of law and the public availability of reliable health care data. In what follows, I describe what appear to be some of the main sources of antagonism toward market-based health care, and then look to ways that such worries can be addressed by those concerned with the future of Chinese health care.

2 Antagonism Toward Markets in Health Care

If markets are as efficacious in producing the multifarious and important economic and moral benefits as suggested, then one might justifiably wonder why markets (especially in health care) fill so many individuals with deep-seated feelings of discomfort and/or outright hostility. Any attempt exhaustively to explain these ubiquitous reactions in a brief paper would no doubt fail miserably, but three of the more prominent general reasons can be identified.

2.1 *Strong Identification of Markets with Particular Instantiations of Market-like Entities that Lack the Requisite Supporting Institutions*

One of the main sources of confusion and ultimately antagonism about markets stems from a failure to remember a basic insight drawn from the teachings of Socrates – namely, that a concept is not identical with any of the particular (or related) instantiations of that concept. Indeed, were many critics of the "market" to engage in a dialogue with Socrates what they surely would be told is, "I have heard what you think about this or that particular market-like institution, but what is it that you find troubling about markets themselves?"

Now, my intention is not to defend Socratic dialectic or any metaphysical thesis regarding forms, but simply to point out an obvious way in which persons can subtly fall victim to fallacious reasoning by failing to disambiguate the economic concept of a market from the many (undoubtedly) poor imitations of the market that abound in the world. In fact, most of the features of markets that persons find most problematic are only accidentally, and not essentially, related to markets. More specifically, and with more careful analysis, the criticisms people levy against the market almost always (1) would be more properly directed against the political or legal institutional frameworks in which markets operate, or (2) can be traced to the circumstance that a market has not sufficiently matured to the point where spontaneously arising solutions have been given a chance to succeed. For example, Hernando de Soto (2000) has convincingly argued that many failures attributed to attempts at market reforms in countries outside the industrial West stem not from markets, but from the fact that the underlying system of property rights is informal, fragmented, and extralegal. In countries where property is governed by formal and unified legal systems, these problems are rare and minor by comparison. When one encounters problems that are purported to be the product of market failures, one would do best to consider first whether the problems would best be addressed by changing bad laws, public policy, etc. or by encouraging the development of corrective market mechanisms.

2.2 Viewing Health Care as Distinct from Other Commodities

Undoubtedly, a second significant reason why so many people feel squarely opposed to health care being delivered through the channels of free markets and private health care institutions is that they have accepted the prevailing moral and political paradigm that health care is somehow unlike other goods and services that are straightforwardly viewed as commodities. Instead, as this paradigm instructs, health care is special; it has the ontological status of an object of a right rather than an article of trade. The distinctive ontological status of health care is often derived from a belief that health care is a basic good and essential for securing equality of opportunity; leaving it vulnerable to market forces would only exacerbate the difficulty in realizing good and honoring this principle. Consider, for example, Cherry's (2003) review of various prominent expressions of this view:

> Because health care is a fundamental good, the moral ideals of justice, equality, and community require that the health care system be universal, comprehensive, and equitable in the sharing of benefits and costs (Brock & Daniels, 1994, p. 1189).
>
> It is health care's role in promoting equality of opportunity that makes ensuring access to health care for all a fundamental requirement of justice (Brock, 2001, p. 164).
>
> Health care needs are basic insofar as they promote fair equality of opportunity. Health care for children is especially important in relation to other social goods, because diseases and disabilities inhibit children's capacities to use and develop their talents, thereby curtailing their opportunities (Kopelman, 2001, p. 202).

Needless to say, one would be hard-pressed to find similar expressions regarding coffee tables, sports cars, swimming pools, or any of a vast variety of ordinary commodities. It is not surprising, given the ontological assumptions in place here, to find this paradigm instructing further that the morally appropriate venue for the delivery of health care lies in ostensibly public and/or non-profit channels. Accordingly, health care is then quickly assumed to be, like the objects of other moral, political, or legal rights (and unlike objects such as coffee tables, sports cars, or swimming pools), the kind of thing for which equal distribution is the guiding pattern.

Free markets characterized by loosely connected and spontaneously originating private health care institutions, of course, do not operate either explicitly or implicitly with this type of egalitarian guiding pattern. Moreover, as Nozick (1974, Ch. 7) is famous for pointing out, such markets and institutions actually tend to "upset" patterns of this sort. Genuinely free markets are committed to allowing buyers, sellers, and traders to interact commercially without the constraints of totalizing principles, save that agreements are fulfilled as promised and in accordance with the general rule of law. In such contexts, even persons who found that they were pursuing a set of market interests generally homogeneous with those with whom they interact would most likely find that they do not rank these general interests in a homogeneous fashion. Whatever the outcomes of their interactions under the conditions of free trade, then, material equality is certainly not to be expected.

This is not the place to address in any detail the problems involved with viewing health care as a fundamental entitlement that persons have in virtue of some feature or other. The moral and political dangers of taking this view of health care have been convincingly examined in Engelhardt's paper in this volume (Engelhardt, 2008). Suffice it to say that adopting this perspective involves (1) engaging the monumental task of drawing a clear conceptual and normative line between those medical interventions to which one has a right and those to which one does not (e.g., cosmetic surgery), while also (2) accepting the inevitable lowering of the standard of care that accompanies a robust commitment to extending universal and equal rights to health care, regardless of ability to pay, under conditions of social financial finitude (Goodman, 2005). Whatever else one has to say about these problems, they are certainly rather large bullets to bite.

Simply put, free markets and private health care institutions are fundamentally incongruent with viewing health care as a right to which all persons are entitled. As a consequence, markets are treated as objects of disapprobation by those wedded to this vision of health care.

2.3 *Inflated Confidence in Public and/or Non-profit Systems of Health Care Delivery*

Another prominent reason that no doubt figures into many persons' distaste for health care markets is the belief that such markets are far surpassed by more centralized, public networks in ways ranging from quality of care and moral integrity to scientific and technological excellence. There are at least two motivating considerations to separate out here. The first is a prevalent view that systems as complex and important as those underlying the delivery of health care must have a good deal of central planning and should not be left hostage to the unpredictable outcomes of unruly markets.[2] Without some coherent and all-encompassing vision to unify and provide direction for all the various elements of a health care system, this view suggests, we risk compromising the ideals of justice and quality thought to lie at its very core. The second point consists in a long running strand of thought, at least in the U.S., that working for a non-profit or governmental agency of whatever sort is a strong indicator that one is genuinely committed to advancing the public interest, untainted by the greed and corruption of for-profit business. Indeed, and more specifically, for many it is simply unfathomable to think that health care practitioners working for private profit could deliver the same quality of care and personal attention as their non-profit, non-private counterparts.[3] Likewise, it is difficult for many to take seriously the idea that such practitioners or the institutions in which they work could maintain strong commitments to moral integrity in the face of the purportedly competing demands of profit. Thus, the objection goes, if one wants better and morally superior health care delivery, then one should be extremely cautious about employing the mechanisms of markets and private health care institutions.

As with the previous two factors underlying market skepticism, this third reason seems misguided both in its criticism of markets and in its inflated confidence in centrally planned and ostensibly public-focused alternatives. While some central planning is often relatively innocuous, the reality of most health care systems is a tendency to move beyond this level to forms of planning with more pernicious outcomes, such as price or wage setting, rationing, and protection of favored interests against the competition generally needed to fuel innovation and cost effectiveness. The cumulative effect of such outcomes is the systematic distortion of the very processes most likely to make efficient and effective use of medical resources. Thus, rather than harnessing the productive and innovative power of relatively unencumbered market forces, while pursuing any wider distributive goals through direct (e.g., income redistribution or subsidized health care) as opposed to indirect (e.g., price fixing) channels, centrally planned health care systems tend to run production and distribution patterns together, thereby compromising the potential of both.

Similarly, it is important to note the fact that, despite popular beliefs to the contrary, an institution's being "public" or "non-profit" is not necessarily positively correlated with its being personal, altruistic, uncorrupted, of high moral integrity, etc. More to the point, when an institution that is "public" or "non-profit" is of any real scale at all, it tends to be highly bureaucratized and thus not centrally characterized by "altruism and personal concern for others" (Cherry, 2003, p. 271). A general point that can be drawn is that as systems for health care delivery grow beyond some critical scale, they inevitably will have something of an impersonal feel about them, regardless of whatever other properties constitute their institutional identity (e.g., public/private, for-profit/non-profit, etc.). Moreover, when public institutional networks for health care delivery take on this impersonal aura, it serves to conceal what would otherwise be regarded as *anti-personal* activities, such as non-transparent rationing and patient queuing. These shortcomings are in addition to the significantly lower levels of productivity and innovation that tend to plague public, governmental, and/or non-profit alternatives to markets. In short, market-based systems for health care delivery are not at a qualitative and/or moral disadvantage when compared with their counterparts (Goodman, 2005).

3 Reconsidering Virtue and Moral Integrity in the Market

In what follows, primary attention will be given to engaging the oft-heard claims that private, for-profit health care delivery (1) corrodes the quality and attentiveness of medical care, the physician-patient relationship, and the professional virtues of medical practitioners, and (2) represents a morally and scientifically inferior alternative to more centralized and rationally planned modes of public delivery. I will argue that these claims overlook the ubiquitous problems and deficiencies of many non-profit or governmental alternatives to private for-profit health care delivery, while simultaneously ignoring or flouting the ways in which genuine profit maximizing strategies require the development and retailing of quality care, professional virtue, and institutional moral integrity.

As I have already argued, market-based systems for health care delivery are not, in principle, at a qualitative and/or moral disadvantage when compared with their counterparts. However, an even stronger claim can be defended here, as the argument contending that private for-profit health care institutions corrode vitally important elements of the health care system can actually be turned on its head. For, upon closer examination, properly functioning and sufficiently mature markets left unencumbered by bad laws or public policy will actually tend to foster a professional health culture that takes seriously and responds genuinely to the needs, desires, and values of its customers (i.e., patients). To begin with, long-term success in the market requires assuring customers that they will be thoughtfully, honestly, and appropriately treated. Virtue in the market is a reliable, long-term, profit-maximizing strategy.[4] Since the market is constituted not by single-instance Prisoner's dilemmas, but rather by long-term dynamic processes, the profitable strategy is to provide customers with the highest satisfaction possible and to strive to attain a good reputation in the marketplace. In the long run, profits are a function of customer satisfaction which is a function of trustworthiness, reliability, and attentiveness to customer needs, wants, and values. That is, profits are a function of long-term commitments to institutional and professional virtues.

Consider, for example, an analogy to something more mundane, such as automotive repair. In this line of business, the name of the game is repeat business and customer referrals of new business. While one could perhaps get by in the short term without attracting such business, it is highly unlikely that long-term growth and profitability can be achieved in their absence. Simply put, there seem to be several basic and necessary conditions that define the good auto mechanic:

(1) A quality job of repairing automobiles,
(2) Within a reasonable price range,
(3) With the reliability promised,
(4) While attending to customer's concerns.

Of course, these conditions are more likely to be realized when mechanics are accountable to the rule of law and not just their own internal standards and commitments. But in the space over and above the rule of law, one can expect to find that those businesses that are profitable in the long run will be those which have best attended to the provision of a quality of service that satisfies customers.

There is no obvious reason why the provision of health care ought to be viewed in a fundamentally different way than the provision of automotive repair. In markets where there is knowledge of the quality of the goods and services provided, competition can arise among providers of goods and services in terms of their trustworthiness, reliability, and attentiveness to customers. The appropriate functioning of health care systems requires both public knowledge of the quality and character of the health care provided and the ability of patients to choose between better and worse quality providers. Furthermore, given the tendencies of governments throughout the world to be overly bureaucratized, private health care and market mechanisms offer advantages for the encouragement of institutional and professional virtue, along with a genuine commitment to high-quality, patient-driven health care. A good example of this insight in practice can be drawn from the successes of alternative mail and package delivery businesses in the U.S. In many ways, the success of companies like FedEx or United Parcel Service (UPS) can be attributed to the overbureaucratization of the U.S. Postal Service and its consequent failures, in addition to their independent commitments to being reliable and trustworthy providers of high-quality delivery services. The key to the nurturing of the integrity of health care institutions and the moral professionalism of physicians is to encourage the availability of good outcome data, so as not only to advantage particular patients, but to give strong incentives for institutional commitments to the quality provision of health care, with attention to the needs and wishes of patients. Here, the rule of law in preventing fraudulent claims is crucial.

Finally, one must note the appropriateness of the development of institutional differences, of particular health care institutions taking on their own moral character. In all markets, tastes and concerns differ. It will be important to recognize that particular health care institutions may very well develop a particular moral vision (e.g., Confucian) for the provision of health care. Such institutional moral identity can naturally draw on local cultural strengths, while providing space for them to give concrete guidance to the commitments and integrity of those particular institutions. Such flourishing of moral diversity, responding to different moral needs and concerns, finds its natural place in market economies with private institutions. All societies and cultures, as they go to the future, will need to examine how, by drawing on their own cultural strengths, the anonymity of the market can lead, paradoxically, to strong commitments to quite particular understandings of moral integrity and to the provision of quality health care through diverse health care institutions.

4 Concluding Remarks: China and the Market

As China looks to health care in the twenty-first century, there are no good reasons for viewing market mechanisms as incompatible with encouraging professional virtues such as trust and moral integrity. First, there are no clear grounds for treating health care services as fundamentally unlike other services that are treated straightforwardly as commodities. Such market-hostile understandings raise unnecessary, and perhaps intractable, conceptual problems, while simultaneously ignoring the realities of social, economic, and medical finitude. Second, although there are grounds to account for a prevailing suspicion of the market, these stem from a failure to appreciate that most defects in the market arise from the absence of appropriate framing institutions such as the rule of law and access to reliable information concerning market outcomes. The latter can be produced by consumer groups, i.e. associations of purchasers of services. The former is more difficult to establish and engrain, as it often requires large-scale changes to existing political attitudes and institutions. Yet there are good reasons for thinking that the extent of China's success or failure with health care markets will ultimately rest, not so much with any putatively inherent properties of markets themselves, but rather on a concomitant commitment to the rule of law as a necessary framing institution. Simply put, there are no reasons to view markets themselves as particularly probable sources of moral malfeasance. Markets (or any alternative productive and distributive mechanism for that matter) depend on law, public policy, and supporting institutions that can achieve rule of law, punish fraud, and root out corrupt practices. Mature markets supported by appropriate institutions should in fact encourage professional and institutional virtue in health care delivery.

Notes

1 The classic works of relevance here are Mandeville's (1988) *The Fable of the Bees: or, Private Vices, Publick Benefits* and Smith's (1981) *An Inquiry into the Nature and Causes of the Wealth of Nations.*

2 Classic critiques of central planning in general are found in von Mises (1936/1981) and Hayek (1948). For an interesting critique of central planning in the macro-allocation of health care, see Meadowcroft's (2003) article on the National Health Service in Great Britain.

3 For examples of such thinking, see Matthews (1998) and Heubel (2000).

4 For more detailed analysis of virtue or ethical behavior as a long-term profit-maximizing strategy, see Engelhardt (1991) and Engelhardt and Rie (1992).

References

Brock, D. (2001). Children's rights to health care. *Journal of Medicine and Philosophy, 26*, 163–178.

Brock, D., & Daniels, N. (1994). Ethical foundations of the Clinton administration's proposed health care system. *Journal of the American Medical Association, 271*, 1189–1196.

Cherry, M. J. (2003). Scientific excellence, professional virtue, and the profit motive: The market and health care reform. *Journal of Medicine and Philosophy,* 28, 259–280.
De Soto, H. (2000). *The Mystery of capital.* New York: Basic Books.
Engelhardt, H. T., Jr. (1991). Virtue for hire: Some reflections on free choice and the profit motive in the delivery of health care. In T. Bole & W. Bondeson (Eds.), *Rights to health care* (pp. 327–353). Dordrecht: Kluwer Academic Publishers.
Engelhardt, H. T., Jr. (2008). China, beware: What American health care has to learn from Singapore. In J. Tao (Ed.), *China: Bioethics, trust, and the challenge of the market* (pp. XXX–XXX). Dordrecht: Springer.
Engelhardt, H. T., Jr., & Rie, M. A. (1992). Selling virtue: Ethics as a profit maximizing strategy in health care delivery. *Journal of Health and Social Policy,* 4, 27–35.
Goodman, J. C. (2005, January 27). Health care in a free society: Rebutting the myths of national health insurance, *Policy Analysis,* 532, 1–26.
Hayek, F. A. (1948). *Individualism and economic order.* Chicago: University of Chicago Press.
Heubel, F. (2000). Patients or customers: Ethical limits of market economy in health care. *Journal of Medicine and Philosophy,* 25, 240–253.
Kopelman, L. (2001). On duties to provide basic health and dental care to children. *Journal of Medicine and Philosophy, 26,* 193–209.
Mandeville, B. (1988). *The fable of the bees: or, private vices, publick benefits* (2 Vols.). F. B. Kaye (Ed.). Indianapolis: Liberty Fund.
Matthews, E. (1998). Is health care a need? *Medicine, Health Care, and Philosophy, 1,* 155–161.
Meadowcroft, J. (2003). The British National Health Service: Lessons from the "socialist calculation Debate." *Journal of Medicine and Philosophy, 28,* 307–326.
Nozick, R. (1974). *Anarchy, state, and Utopia.* New York: Basic Books.
Smith, A. (1981). *An inquiry into the nature and causes of the wealth of nations* (Vols. I and II). In R. H. Campbell & A. S. Skinner (Eds.), *Vol. II of the Glasgow Edition of the Works and Correspondence of Adam Smith.* Indianapolis: Liberty Fund.
von Mises, L. (1936/1981). *Socialism.* J. Kahane (Trans., 2nd English Ed.). Indianapolis: Liberty Fund.

Part V
Looking to the Future of China: Can Confucius Guide the Health Care Market?

On the Reform of Health Care Reform[1]

Ren-Zong Qiu

1 The Debate on the Evaluation of Health Care Reform

The "Evaluation and Recommendations on the Reform of Chinese Health System (Summary[2])" report was recently published by the Center for Development, which is affiliated with the State Council or Central Government. The Report has received divergent comments. However, it is natural that there are different opinions on the report.

I stated at the Jinan Conference that so far we cannot claim that health care reform has been successful; the negative consequences which it has caused have outweighed the positive consequences that it has brought about. As early as two years ago at a meeting to summarize the experiences and lessons of SARS prevention and control, health care reform was criticized for involving "more reform and less health care." Indeed, at the early stage of health care reform, many people had differing opinions on the orientation of health care reform. At a meeting on health care reform and development, many participants criticized the practices that attempted to apply the contract system in agriculture to heath care.[3] However, the former and late Minister of Health did not accept any of these critiques and the meeting parted in bad terms.

Health care reform has already had 20 years of experience. Whether the 20 years of health care reform has been unsuccessful or successful is a value judgment. Indeed, participants of the debate may have different data, and there may be differences between data available to them, but what is more important is the divergence in value judgment. The different evaluations of health care reform originate from the differing expectations and objectives that one has concerning health care reform.

2 Unjust Consequences Caused by Health Care Reform

The consequences caused by health care reform are positive as well as negative. The positive consequences have been mentioned in the Report. Perhaps, it should

---

R.-Z. Qiu
Institute of Philosophy, Chinese Academy of Social Sciences, Beijing, PRC, China
e-mail: rzq@chinaphs.org

J. Tao (ed.), *China: Bioethics, Trust, and the Challenge of the Market*,

© Springer Science+Business Media B.V. 2008

be pointed out that after 20 years of reform, the capacity to diagnose and treat diseases has improved. We now possess technological means more advanced than ever before and we have built many hospitals and institutes, which can be compared with the best in the world. We have also trained a range of young, able professionals and many important clinical institutions all over the country no longer need to rely mainly on support from the government. They not only assume sole responsibility for their profits and costs, but also have surplus of assets, and the income and living standard of medical professionals have greatly improved. This is the original intention of health care reform. However, it has to be admitted that the costs for these achievements is heavy or even tragic, because more people now do not have the resources to see a doctor, and have to wait for death or sell all their property to pay for medical costs, which often results in the family breaking up or plunging into poverty (Zhou 2003).

A poll conducted by the Center for Social Services and published in *Chinese Youth Daily* shows that 90% of respondents were unsatisfied with the health care changes made in the last ten years. It may be argued that this can be used as evidence to evaluate health care services. However, because 90% of patients expressed satisfaction concerning health care services in some surveys conducted by the hospitals themselves, the credibility of these surveys has to be greatly discounted (He, 2005). For us, it is necessary to look at the data published by the authoritative institutes.

The Third National Survey on Health Care Services published in the end of 2004 shows that 48.9% of Chinese did not see a doctor when they fell ill, and 29.6% who would have been admitted to the hospital did not enter it (Yan, 2005). This survey also shows that in the past five years the average income of inhabitants in urban and rural areas increased by 8.9% and 2.4%, respectively, but that the health care payout increased by 13.5% and 11.8%, respectively. According to the data in the "Summary of 2005 China's Health Care Statistics", published by the Ministry of Health, among the total health care costs, the health care payout by the Government decreased to 17.2% from 36.2%, and the payout by the society decreased to 27.3% from 42.6%, but individual payout dramatically increased in 2000 to 55.5% from 21.2%, and further increased to 60% in 2001 (Zhang, 2005). Table 1 shows the percentage of health care costs afforded by the Chinese government in comparison with other countries in 2000:

The percentage afforded by the Chinese government in total health care costs shows that the government has been withdrawing from the health care field and avoiding its responsibility to provide health care. This cannot be ethically justified. It is often criticized that many of the problems in health care now are caused by

Table 1 The part of total health care costs afforded by the government in different countries in 2000

Developed countries	73.00%
Countries in transition	70.00%
Least developed countries	55.50%
Other developing countries	57.20%
China (mainland)	39.40%

Source: *Health News*, July 1, 2005

putting priority on efficiency and neglecting fairness when implementing health care reform. This critique is correct. However, the data also shows that the consequence of only focusing on efficiency and neglecting fairness in policy orientation is that there is no efficiency as well as fairness.

In respect to fairness:

1. Unfairness in financing: The total amount of national health care expenditures was CNY 54.6 billion yuan;[4] the central government only provided CNY 3.543 billion or 6.5%.
2. Unfairness in universal coverage: In urban areas, the percentage of those employees who enjoy basic medical insurance amounts to 5.6%; those who enjoy the public medical services, 4.0%; those who enjoy labor insurance, 4.6%;[5] those who buy commercial medical insurance, 1%; and those who have no medical insurance at all is about 44.8%. In rural areas the proportion of those who participate in collective medical care amounts to 9.5%; those in various social medical insurance, 3.1%; those who buy commercial medical insurance, 8.3%; and those who have no medical insurance at all, 79.1%. Table 2 shows that the coverage rate of health care has been decreasing year after year in urban and rural areas:
3. Unfairness in the use of health services: either the patients have no money to pay for health services, or they are induced to use excessive services by providers, which may amount to 20–60% of total health care expenditures. Reasonable prescriptions only amount to 2% of total prescriptions. The proportion of costs for repeated and/or irrelevant examinations among the medical costs paid by inpatients and outpatients increased from 28% in 1990 to 36.7% in 2002 (Jin, 2005).

Health statistics show that while the total population is increasing, the number of inpatients in clinics and hospitals as well is decreasing. Total medical costs already account for about 5% of GDP, but almost half of people with illnesses do not go to see a doctor. How is this efficient? (*Health News*, July 1, 2005)

It is an indisputable fact that people complain that it is too expensive and too difficult to see a doctor. Not all people understand the meaning of these two sentences. Since the founding of the People's Republic of China, there was never such complaint until the average GDP *per capita* reached US $1,000. Does it deserve serious consideration and reflection?

Table 2 Medical insurance coverage rates of inhabitants in urban areas and rural areas

Year	Inhabitants in Urban Areas	Inhabitants in Rural Areas
1993	70.0%	5.8%
1998	49.8%	4.7%
2003	43.0%	3.1%

Source: *Health News*, July 1, 2005

3 Possible Refutations to the Unjust Consequences of Health Care Reform

One of the possible refutations of the negative consequences brought about by health care reform may be that the inequality of enjoying health care is not unjust or unfair. In general, inequality is not equated with injustice. The well-off buy cars and the worst-off buy bicycles. This is not always unjust. However, if the well-off can pay for heart surgeries and the worst-off can only wait for death helplessly, then this is unjust in the sense that both of them have a right to life and health care if the condition is curable. In the last 20 years, the priority put on efficiency has brought about a lot of unfair and unjust things, such as the widening of the gap between the well-off and the worst-off (Marchand and Wikler 2002).

The second refutation is that paying for health care should be an individual or personal responsibility. It has been stated that a person's illness is caused either by her/his unhealthy behavior, or by unfortunate exposure to pathogenic factors. So each individual should be responsible for her/his health or disease. However, individual responsibility only plays a marginal role in health or disease, as Wikler argued (Wikler, 2004). The health or disease of a given individual depends on many factors which cannot be controlled by the individual. There is a sense that health or disease is socially determined. Individuals who are working at a workplace where the concentration of many poisonous materials exceed health standards, fall ill in many cases. Even though some of them fell ill because of their unhealthy behavior, it is also unlikely to be her/his individual responsibility to pay for health care since they are not responsible for falling ill. Falling ill is often related to poverty and unavailability of information. Because of poverty, they have to buy food from cheaper free markets which are often ill managed and loosely monitored by the government, and then they fall ill from eating bad food. In many cases, medical information is not available to individuals and the programs of TV stations owned by the central government or provincial/municipal governments are filled with false, fabricated medical advertisements. The most fundamental medical information is rarely provided. Should those who fall ill after following what has been advertised be responsible for their disease?

The third possible refutation is that patients cannot afford their medical costs because their income is too low and this is not related to health reform. Yes, the fact is that individual income (price of the labor force) is lower than the value of the labor force. According to the statistics, state financial income increased to CNY 2,600 billion yuan in 2004 from CNY 1,300 billion yuan in 2000, but the proportion of employees' wages in GDP decreased to 12% in 2003 from 16% in 1989 (Yu, 2005). Many enterprises are engaged in absolute surplus value reproduction, and make their profits by depressing or skimping the wages for labor force reproduction, so that the entrepreneurs do not have to use science and technology or improve the management for survival in the market competition. Self-labeled socialist and Marxist officials are indifferent to this exploitation, and trade unions do not fight for workers' interests at all. This depressing outcome is unfair, and its consequences are serious. One of the consequences is that the economy always depends on the foreign market, and that the demands in the domestic market are impotent for a long time. The difficulty of seeing a doctor because of a lack of income is also unfair.

The fourth possible refutation is that the original intention of health care reform is to lessen the government's burden, and to enable the government to reduce expenditures spent on hospitals and other health care institutions, or even for the government to completely withdraw from the health care field. Health care reform should be deemed successful according to this criterion. This refutation implies that the different evaluations of heath care reform depend on the different expectations or objectives of health care reform. What follows is our discussion of these issues, such as what objectives should health care reform achieve? Why it is wrong to view reducing the government's expenditures or even withdrawing the government from the health care field as the objectives of health care reform?

4 The Benchmarks of the Health Care Reform

From the very beginning of health care reform in China, reducing the government's burden has been seen as the objective or one of major objectives for this reform, and the objectives *comme il faut* have been ignored. The objectives *comme il faut* are those objectives based on ethical considerations: what ethically justified objectives should health care reform achieve? There have been different answers to this question from the very beginning of health care reform.

Norman Daniels, an expert in health policy and a professor at Harvard University and his colleagues have been working on the benchmarks of health care reform (Daniels, 2000). At first they proposed the following benchmarks as criteria to evaluate health care reform in a country as being either successful or unsuccessful:

— Does it reduce barriers to access to public health measures and medical services?
— Does it provide healthcare services appropriate to the needs of the population?
— Does it distribute the burdens of paying for health protection fairly?
— Does the reform promote clinical and administrative efficiency?
— Does it make institutions publicly accountable for their decisions?
— How does it affect the choices people can exercise?

These benchmarks, that is, accessibility, responsiveness to needs, fairly distributing burdens, efficiency, accountability and choice enlarging, can be ethically justified on the basis of major ethical principles. I do not think it is necessary for me to provide detailed arguments here, because it is somehow self-evident. Only for the first benchmark, reducing various financial and non-financial barriers to access to public health measures and medical services is seen as a very important step to reach universal coverage for all citizens. We are not able to achieve this ideal overnight, however. It is reasonable to require increasing the access and enlarging the coverage after each reform. It is a shame that no matter what positive evaluation of health care reform is made, as the date above shows, it is an indisputable fact that during the 20 years of health care reform, the financial and non-financial barriers to access to public health measures and medical services have increased and the coverage of health insurance has been reduced.

Professors Norman Daniels and John Bryant worked with colleagues in Columbia, Mexico, Pakistan and Thailand to further revise the benchmarks applied in developing countries. The revised version of the benchmarks is as follows (Daniels, 2000):

Benchmark 1: Intersectoral public health: The rationale for this benchmark is that social determinants and other risk factors "upstream" from the point of health-care delivery to affect population health, including basic nutrition, housing, environmental factors, education and health education, public safety and violence reduction. The first criterion in this benchmark asks for estimates of the degree to which a population benefits from reductions in exposure to various risk factors as a result of the reforms under consideration. The second criterion calls for developing an information infrastructure needed to measure and monitor health inequalities and to carry out research about the most effective ways to reduce these. The third criterion evaluates reforms for their coverage across sectors and their involvement with communities and vulnerable groups in these efforts.

Benchmark 2: Financial barriers to equitable access: Fairness requires reducing financial and non-financial barriers to access to needed services. Benchmark 2 recognizes the large "informal," non-taxable employment sector in many developing countries (often 60–90% of the population) and encourages a long-term strategy aimed at moving as much of the population as possible into the formal sector and then into insurance schemes that can be built on broadly based general tax revenues, social security payments or employer-based contributions. Benchmark 2 also specifies interim goals in both sectors, and encourages reforms to specify a basic package of services that all will receive by a specific target date, and then to improve that package over time.

Benchmark 3: Non-financial barriers to equitable access: The first criterion evaluates reforms according to the measures they take to address the poor distribution of drugs, supplies, facilities and personnel. The second, third, and fourth criteria address respectively gender barriers, cultural barriers and discrimination by race, religion, class, sexual orientation, disease, including stigmatisation of groups receiving public care.

Benchmark 4: Comprehensiveness of benefits: The underlying rationale is that all people, regardless of class or ethnicity or gender, have comparable health needs and there are similar social obligations to meet these. Inequalities in the coverage and quality of care reduce the fairness of systems. All effective and needed services should be deemed affordable, by all needed providers without categorical exclusions.

Benchmark 5: Equitable financing: The fundamental idea is that financing medical services, as opposed to access, should be according to the ability to pay. Three main sources of funding are involved in most systems: tax-based revenues, insurance premiums and out-of-pocket payments. Tax-based schemes are more equitable if their structure is more progressive. Premium-based schemes are more equitable if they are community-rated, rather than risk-rated. Risk-rating shifts the burden to those with a higher risk of illness. The same inequity is involved in out-of-pocket contributions in both tax-based and premium-based systems.

Benchmark 6: Efficacy, efficiency, and quality of care: The rationale is that, all other things being equal, a system that gets more value for money in the use of its resources is fairer to those in need. Distributive justice and fairness are important because resources are always limited. A key criterion in Benchmark 6 is primary health care for community-based delivery. Reforms aimed at improving primary care must assure appropriate training, incentives, resource allocation and community participation in decisions affecting delivery. Emphasis is placed on a population focus and on the need for the integration of different parts of the health system.

Benchmark 7: Administrative efficiency: Benchmark 7 seeks efficiency in the management of the healthcare system. Addressing these problems, however, also requires greater accountability, including transparency.

Benchmark 8: Democratic accountability and empowerment: The rationale for including accountability is that health systems are responsible for the improvement of population health in an equitable manner, and those affected by decisions and policies that affect their well-being in such fundamental ways must have an understanding of and ultimate control over that system.

Benchmark 9: Patient and provider autonomy: This benchmark may raise questions such as the following: How important is autonomy or choice? In some market-based approaches, informed choice is necessary if quality is to be improved and true preferences met. But how much choice should be given and what kinds of choices? Similarly, provider autonomy is much sought after by professionals, but is often seen by planners as an obstacle to the efficient use of services.

Regrettably enough, although Professors Norman Daniels and John Bryant tried to involve Chinese officials or scholars into the work on developing benchmarks for health care reform, their invitation was denied.

Which approach to health care reform can be justified ethically? Those benchmarks listed above, or the aim of reducing the burdens from the government, or the aim of the government of completely withdrawing from the health care field as some economists proposed? As I argued in an article (Qiu, 2003) titled "Ethical and Policy Issues Raised in the SARS Epidemic," the important role of health care in national economy is not well understood; this non-understanding may be the error of all previous governments. Concerning the relationship between health care and national economy, people only seem to recognize the dependence of health care upon the national economy, but do not recognize the contribution of health care to the national economy. In this situation, people chose efficiency of administering health care, but ignore fairness. Of course, we may focus on solving the efficiency issue in one period and focus on solving the fairness issue in the next period. However, by no means, can we ignore each of these issues. Economists may focus on the efficiency issue. However, those economists who do not care about fairness at all may be called outdated economists or halfway economists (Qiu, 2003). As the experiences of health care reform in China shows, there is no efficiency without fairness.

5 The Role of the Market in Health Care

Among the people who agree on the issue of the failure of health care reform there is still disagreement on the cause of this basic non-success: is it because of market-orientation of health care reform or is it because of the distortion of the market in health care?

For Dr. Frederic Fransen it is a misunderstanding to ascribe the greedy behaviors in the health care market to the market (Fransen, 2005). He cites Friedrich Hayek (Hayek, 1948) in claiming that such a view fundamentally misunderstands the basic problem of economics and the actual role played by markets. According to Hayek, the basic problem of economic organization is how to rapidly transmit complex information about changes in conditions affecting supply and demand to those who can use it to adjust their production or consumption. How do they communicate this information? The answer, Hayek argues, is by means of prices. The price mechanism, according to Hayek, is really an ingenious device, discovered accidentally by man, to transmit vast amounts of information about economic conditions to those who can make use of it. What role do markets play? First, markets are the places – physical or virtual – in which people come together to engage in exchange based upon their desires, given a set of relative prices. This is a very delicate process, because those desires are often affected by the prices themselves, so markets provide a very intricate feedback mechanism to help people maximize their ability to fulfill their (varied) desires. In order for the price mechanism to convey accurate information, these prices – and the exchanges that take place based upon them – need to be arrived at voluntarily. In any real market, they can and will only take place if each party to an exchange believes that the object he receives is of more value to him than the one which he is offering in trade. Thus, markets are places in which people come together to transmit information by trading things they consider of less value for those they consider to be of more value. At the end of every voluntary exchange, although nothing new is produced, both parties have increased their wealth as they understand it.

Health care services as a commodity can be exchanged according to the market mechanism, as Hayek described. The market where the information conveyed is intentionally distorted or fraudulent, the exchange is not voluntary, and after this exchange only one party increases its wealth, and the other even does not know if its wealth is increased, is not a real market, but a distorted market. Producers of goods, services, and capital meet with consumers to extort as much profit out of them as possible so it is not the fault of the market. This view is very popular. In an article "Market Is Not the Scapegoat for Unaffordability" (Huang, 2005), the author suggests that those public non-profit hospitals are "deformed." On one hand they provide services to consumers-patients in the market and make profits. On the other hand, they emphasize that they are public and non-profit hospitals, and plead to the government to increase their budget. They enjoy the privilege of exemption from taxation and make excessive profits. So the market they participate in is not a real market, but rather a distorted one.

How then can we build a real market in health care? Or is it even possible to build a real market as described by Hayek? Even if we build a real market, does it solve the problem of being too expensive and too difficult to see a doctor? Except for the interest group that profits from it, nobody defends overtly this distorted market. The majority recognizes that this market of health care is a "deformed" one. But nobody suggests that it can be treated or cured. In my opinion, the "deformed" market brings too much harm to many patients and their families. In the exchange, a few people increase their wealth, but too many people are deprived of their wealth, and even life. Whether those who claim the way out is to build a real market, or those who claim the way out is for the government to play a leading role, both may agree that decisive measures have to be taken to end this deformed or distorted market. However, can a real market that is pervasive in all fields of health care as described by Hayek be built?

I do not think that the market can solve the problems we are facing in health care. I pointed out in *Bioethics* (Qiu, 1987, pp. 284–287) that basic medical and preventive measures should be ensured, and those measured should be enlarged with socio-economic and scientific-technological development, and the commercialization of health care is not preferable as it is not compatible with the nature of health care. However, it is also not a good system where the state is only provider. I agree with George Soros when he said that the market is the best of the worst mechanisms of resources allocation (Qiu, 2003). He followed the evaluation of democracy made by Sir Winston Churchill to the effect that democracy is the best of the worst political system. Simply put, neither democracy nor the market is perfect. They are better than any other system, but they also have shortcomings. The market is not able to guarantee social justice, provide non-profit preventive and medical services, provide health care to the vulnerable, and protect the environment, etc. The government should be responsible for these things.

Actually, many scholars have already discussed these issues. Professor Du (Du, 2005) pointed out that the marketization of medical care would force the hospitals to pursue profits and move away from their real goals; the commercialization of medical care would dramatically increase medical costs and impose heavy burdens to the state, institutions and individuals; the commercialization of medical care would waste resources, and cause an inequitable allocation of resources; the commercialization of medical care would weaken prevention and primary health care; and the market and the commercialization of health care services would cause corruption. Other scholars (e.g. Gong 2005, Liu, 2005) also claim that the characteristics of medical care consist of being a public good, high asymmetry of information, randomness of risks and rigidity of consumption, etc.

I would like to add that the market is formed under certain economic conditions. For example, only when people have money in their pockets can they be a partner in the exchange. However, many peasants in China have no money, and some even have debt after working hard for one year. If they cannot become a partner in the exchange, how can the market solve their health care needs? Clean water delivery and waste management in countryside, public toilets and garbage treatment in cities, and vaccine inoculation for the huge number of children – all of these cannot be relied upon the market to provide. In Hong Kong, one of the most mature market in the world, medical authority recently decided that those who possess usable property under 20,000 HK dollars can enjoy free medical care at public hospitals, and those who possess usable property more than 600,000 HK dollars cannot get any subsidies in medical care (Huang, 2005). The decision shows that medical care for the worst off cannot be provided for by the market, that the market is not willing to provide such care, and that it cannot do it well.

Furthermore, there is some connection between the real market and the distorted market. It is related with characteristics of health care: in the physician-patient relationship, the patient is in a vulnerable position in which patient and physician are not equal in their possession of information or knowledge. The nature of this relationship imposes on the physician the duty to help on the one hand, and create a possibility for the physician to exploit the patient on the other hand. You can find numerous cases of this exploitation in the health care market all over the world. It is why Chinese ancient doctors warn physicians "before we treat the patient, we treat our own heart first" (Liu Fang) and "The way of practicing medicine is that we have to rectify ourselves first and then treat illness with medicine" (Anonymous). The best measure to protect patients is to separate a physician's income from a patient's payment, although this would be incompatible with the market.

One more question that we have to answer is whether it is unnecessary for the market to play some role in the provision of health care. If we assume that the market has its role in health care, then what is the relationship between the market mechanism and the government's role?

Professor H. Tristram Engelhardt, Jr. (Engelhardt, 2005) has argued for the necessity of the market in health care on the basis of some assumptions. He argued that in order to confront the challenges of health care financing, we must embrace a system that:

1. Promises to all some basic health care, but not the best care,
2. Recognizes that health care will be unequally available, while
3. Making patients and their families recognize the cost of these health care services.

Then he proposed that a health care system should have one or more of the following sorts of providers:

1. Private for-profit providers, including individual practitioners, hospitals, and corporations formed to provide health care;
2. Private not-for-profit providers, including individual practitioners, hospitals, and corporations formed to provide health care;
3. Governmental entities, including hospitals and health care systems that, though governmental, are local and may still compete among each other as well as with private for-profit and not-for-profit providers in attracting patients and physicians;
4. Unified governmental systems that provide health care.

Engelhardt's proposal seems to be not so different from that of many scholars in China: reserve some room for the market in health care. He suggests promising all some basic health care, but not the best care, and unifying governmental systems that provide health care. This precludes the marketizaton of health care. The issue that remains is what kind of role the market and the government should play in health care. Which should be dominant: the market or the government?

The conclusion is that health care reform needs to reform. The first thing in the agenda of the reform of health care reform is to develop benchmarks for health care reform on the basis of our experiences and lessons of the past 20 years of reform and in reference to work that has been done by scholars from other countries.

Notes

1 This paper is an expanded version of my presentation at the Conference on Health Care, Market and Confucian Morality, in Jinan on June 27–28, 2005. The summary of "Evaluation and Recommendations on the Reform of Chinese Health System" has not been read.

2 The author has not had the chance to read its full text so far.

3 The title of my presentation at this meeting was "Health Care from Ethical Perspective" in which I argued that "although the contract system in hospitals may bring about some short-term benefits, but in the long run the costs would outweigh the benefits", and that "health care, education, public security and defense are to safeguard the basic rights of citizens, and cannot be commercialized". I also argued that "only 3% of government expenditures are allocated to health care and letting medical professionals improve their life standards by themselves is unethical". Also, a "two-tiered system is practical: national health insurance only covers basic health needs, apart from some commercial hospitals can be approved to run." (*The Proceedings of the Symposium on Health Care and Development*, Beijing: Chinese Health Economics Press, November 16–18, 1998, pp. 61–62.)

4 One US dollar exchanged to eight Chinese yuan.

5 Since the founding of the People's Republic of China, two systems were established: public medical insurance for employees working at the state institutions, which provides them with free medical care as the payments came from the government; and labor insurance for employees working at state factories where they too, enjoy free medical care, but the payment comes from factories. Both of these systems have been in bankruptcy as of late.

References

Center for Development, State of Council. (2005). *Evaluation and recommendations on the reform of Chinese health system* (Summary). [On-line]. Available: www.sohu.com.

Chi, H. (2005, July 14). Public health strategy in the late 20th century: Same mistake was committed by the East and West. *Southern Weekend*, B16.

Daniels, N. (2000). Benchmarks of fairness for healthcare reform: A policy tool for developing countries. *Bulletin of the World Health Organization, 78*(6), 1–31.

Du, Z. (2005, June 27–28). *Establishing a humanistic health care market*. International Conference on Health Care Services, Markets, and the Confucian Moral Tradition, Jinan.

Engelhardt, H. T., Jr. (2005, June 27–28). *Why the United States have had difficulties: Recognizing the importance of its private health care sector*. International Conference on Health Care Services, Markets, and the Confucian Moral Tradition, Jinan.

Fransen, F. J. (2005, June 27–28). *Markets, trust, and the nurturing of a culture of responsibility: Implications for health care policy*. International Conference on Health Care Services, Markets, and the Confucian Moral Tradition, Jinan.
Gong, S. M. (2005, June 8). Marketization cannot solve the problem "Medical care too expensive". *China's Youth.*
Hayek, F. (1948). The use of knowledge in society. In *Individualism and economic order* (pp. 77–91). Chicago: University of Chicago press.
He, T. Q. (2005, September 1). Two different kinds of "Degree of satisfactoriness". *Health News*, p. 4.
Huang, B. (2005, June 8). "Market" is not the scapegoat for medical care too expensive. *Health News.*
Jin, Y. H. (2005, September 2). How to contain excessive treatment? *Health News*, pp. 3–6.
Liu, H. P. (2005) "Marketization" is contradictory with guiding role by the government. *Health News*, p. 4.
Marchand, S., & Wikler, D. (2002). Equality and the distribution of health. In J. Tao (Ed.), *Cross-cultural perspectives on the (Im)possibility of global bioethics*. Dordrecht: Kluwer Academic Publishers, Inc.
Qiu, R. Z. (1987). *Bioethics*. Shanghai: Shanghai People's Press.
Qiu, R. Z. (1998, November 16–18). Health care from ethical perspective. *The proceedings of the symposium on health care and development* (pp. 61–62). Beijing: Chinese Health Economics Press.
Qiu, R. Z. (2003). Ethical and policy issues raised in SARS epidemic in China. *Studies in Dialectics of Nature*, *6*, 1–5.
Wikler, D. (2004). Personal and social responsibility for health. In S. Anand, F. Peter, & A. Sen (Eds.), *Public Health, Ethics, and Equity* (pp. 109–134). Oxford University Press.
Yan, L. X. (2005, January 12). Health care reform in urban areas: The government should play its role. *Health News.*
Yu, W. (2005, June 20). The deviation of labor force from value increasingly serious. *International Finance Newspaper.*
Zhang, R. (2005, July, 1). On the reform of health care system. *Health News*, p. 7.
Zhou, Y. L. (2003). *Fairness, efficiency and economic growth: A study in health care financing transitional China*. Wuhan: Wuhan Press.

Is Singapore's Healthcare System Morally Problematic?

A Philosophical Analysis

Justin Ho*

1 Introduction

Any country that wishes to maintain a government financed healthcare system, which aims to provide some degree of healthcare, must address the problem of rising costs. If the government chooses to increase its expenditures on health care to meet rising costs, this leads to one or more of the following undesirable consequences:

(1) increasing taxes to cover the rising health care costs
(2) diverting money from other important programs to cover rising health care costs
(3) incurring debt in order to avoid increasing taxes and/or diverting money from other programs

The government can also elect not to spend more money to fund the public health care system and simply cut back on the amount of health care that it subsidizes. However, if the government is morally obligated to fund or provide a certain level of health care for its citizens, the decision to curtail expenditures may be unacceptable.

The health care system of Singapore has recently received attention from certain policy makers, largely because the rising costs of health care have become a pressing issue for many countries. Singapore's healthcare system was ranked first when compared to Canada, the United States, the United Kingdom, Switzerland, Germany, Australia and South Africa in a 2001 study conducted by the Canadian health economist, Cynthia Ramsay, which ranked health care systems based on quality, access to care and cost (Ramsay, 2001). In 2005, the World Health Organization ranked Singapore number 6 out of 191 countries on overall health system performance (World Health Organization, 2005). What drew considerable attention was Singapore's ability to achieve these lofty rankings while managing to limit government spending on health care expenditures through patient financing and government controls. A comparison of Singapore's health care expenditures with

J. Ho
Department of Philosophy, Rice University
e-mail: justinho@rice.edu

* Assistant Managing Editor of the *Journal of Medicine and Philosophy*.

J. Tao (ed.), *China: Bioethics, Trust, and the Challenge of the Market*,
© Springer Science+Business Media B.V. 2008

countries that provide free basic inpatient and outpatient care to all its citizens like the United Kingdom and Canada; with countries that provide free basic inpatient and outpatient care to the medically indigent and the elderly like the United States; and with countries the subsidize the vast majority of inpatient care like Hong Kong, shows that Singapore's government spends considerably less than these countries (See Chart A, B, C, D in the Appendix). This has led some analysts to argue that Singapore's health care system should be used as a model for health care reform (Tucci, 2004). Nevertheless, others have countered by arguing that the system would fail to achieve these results in larger countries or that a more accurate statistical analysis would show that Singapore's system does produce the results that Ramsay and others have claimed (World Bank, 2003).

This chapter will not debate such issues as they fall primarily in the area of health care policy. Rather this chapter will focus more on a number of moral criticisms that have been raised against Singapore's health care system. In particular, attention will be devoted to the moral criticisms contained in Michael T. Barr's (2001) often-cited paper "Medical Savings Accounts in Singapore: A Critical Inquiry" as many persons are likely to find Barr's claims to be convincing. The goal will not be to defend Singapore's health care system against Barr's criticisms, but rather to analyze these criticisms from a philosophical perspective to show what philosophical assumptions and views must be held if Barr's arguments are to have any teeth.

The structure of this chapter is as follows: Section 2 outlines the central features of Singapore's healthcare system; Section 3 addresses Barr's criticisms; Section 4 highlights the philosophical assumptions and views that one must affirm in order for Barr's criticisms to be valid.

2 The Central Features of Singapore's Health Care System

The Singapore health care system is comprised of both a public and a private health care system. Most people who use the private health care system pay for health care themselves, which is why it can be classified as a patient financed health care system (See Chart C & D in the Appendix). A patient seeking inpatient care is classified by the government based on income and/or willingness to pay for healthcare. There are six classes: A1, A2, B1 (air-conditioned), B1 (non- air-conditioned), B2 and C. Only classes A1, A2 and B1 (air-conditioned) are available in private hospitals, which charge patients 100% of costs. However, patients residing in government hospitals may pay as little as 19% of the total costs depending on how they are classified; the rest of the costs are subsidized by the government, which pays for these costs through taxation.

In addition to this classification scheme, there are three central institutional components to Singapore's health care system: a mandatory savings plan (Medisave), a low cost, catastrophic health insurance scheme (Medishield and Eldershield), and a welfare scheme (Medifund). Medisave is run through the Central Provident Fund (CPF), a mandatory social security savings scheme to which both employers and employees contribute. Currently, employees contribute around 20% of their income to the CPF account each month and employers contributes around 13% of their employees' salary to the account.[1] The CPF savings generate interest at market-related rates for their members annually and contributions are tax free and become part of one's estate after death. Savings can also be transferred to family members. Part of the contribution to the CPF (roughly 6–8% of one's salary, depending on one's age) is placed in a Medisave account; a savings account intended to be primarily used to pay for health care costs.

There are number of restrictions on how patients may use their Medisave accounts. To avoid a premature depletion of a patient's Medisave account, caps are placed on the amount a patient can pay using this account. If one chooses a ward that charges more than the standard rates, one must fund these expenditures either privately or using Medishield. Medisave can also be used to pay for certain types of outpatient services. However, the vast majority of outpatient services must be paid for out-of-pocket. Further, patients who have insufficient savings in their Medisave accounts to pay for health care costs may only use future contributions to pay for certain procedures.

Medishield is a low cost, catastrophic health insurance scheme intended to help Medishield members pay for hospitalization costs when Medisave accounts are not sufficient. Medishield also sets limits on the costs for which it will pay. Costs that exceed these limits must be paid for out of pocket. After surpassing a deductible, Medishield will pay for 80% of the costs above the deductible. Eldershield is a basic insurance plan, designed to help cover the expenses of all Singaporeans and Permanent Residents reaching 40 years of age and who have CPF accounts, against severe disability or illness due to old age. Eldershield helps by giving monthly cash handouts and taking care of out-of-pocket expenses. This plan, which has relatively low premiums deductible from the Medisave account, is provided by two companies (Great Eastern Life and NTUC Income). While all workers must contribute part of their income to Medisave, purchasing Medishield and Eldershield is optional.

Finally, Medifund is an endowment fund established by the Singapore government, which helps to pay the health care expenditures of the medically indigent, those persons who are unable to pay for their own medical expenses despite government subsidies. Eligibility for Medifund is assessed by medical social workers on a case-by-case basis.

3 Barr's Criticisms

Barr in his paper raises three substantial, moral criticisms against Singapore's health care system. All of these criticisms arise from measures taken by Singapore's government to control government spending on health care. The first of these criticisms is leveled against the fact that Singapore's government has implemented policies to curb government spending on health care. Singapore has (1) regulated the introduction of technology and medical specialists in government hospitals; (2) introduced a predetermined rate of subsidy for these institutions; (3) ensured that the number of specialists number no more than 40% of the medical profession (1, 2, and 3 are reported in a document by the Ministry of Health entitled "Report of the Cost Review Committee-Response of the Ministry of Health, 1999"); (4) introduced price caps on all medical services delivered in government hospitals (Low, 1998) and (5) restricted the number of government hospital beds (Massaro & Wong, 1995).

Barr seems to argue that all of these controls should be viewed as problematic because they severely limit personal autonomy. As he puts it:

> Singapore's record of keeping its health costs low is attributable primarily to *heavy handed* government control of both inputs and outputs. . .Unfortunately, the *negative features* of government control and rationing are intrinsic features of what is otherwise a laudable achievement: the building of a modern low-cost health system that works satisfactorily for most people most of the time (my italics) (p. 710).

> For most of the population, the cost of moving outside the parameters set by the 3Ms [Medisave, Medishield, and Medifund] (for instance by having a fourth baby) is prohibitive. Far from allowing an open market, the government even regulates the number of doctors and specialists with the stated purpose of dampening demand for healthcare (p. 723).

Barr appears to be arguing that such controls greatly restrict the range of choices that many Singaporeans can make and in some cases persons are prevented from making decisions that are central to promoting their conception of a good life. For instance, because Medishield and Medisave cannot be used to pay for assisted reproduction, persons whose central values include having a family are prevented from pursuing such goals if they lack adequate funds. Or more significantly, those who need dialysis or AIDS medication are prevented from pursuing whatever projects come from an extended life if they lack adequate funds.

Barr does note that persons, whose autonomy is limited, are primarily from the middle and poorer classes. This follows because as long as persons can pay for health care services, they can receive as much health care as they desire. Barr's first criticism then can be summarized as follows:

> Criticism 1: Singapore's Health care system is problematic because of the limits it places on the autonomy of persons in the middle and lower classes.

Barr also criticizes how Singapore's health system rations the number of health care services that can be paid for through Medisave and Medishield. For instance, patients who have insufficient savings in their Medisave account to pay for health care costs cannot use future contributions to pay for certain life prolonging procedures, such as dialysis, radio-therapy, chemotherapy, and AZT treatment. Further, Medisave and Medishield cannot be used to cover the costs for procedures that Barr regards as basic and to which persons have a legitimate moral claim to:

> Although the government is committed to ensuring the provision of "basic health care" for the population, it is unembarrassed about excluding particular procedures from that definition. For instance, Medisave cannot be used to cover maternity ward and associated costs beyond a third child, nor long-term hospital care (Tan & Chew, 1997) and Medishield does not cover a wide range of conditions including congenital abnormalities, cosmetic surgery, maternity charges, abortion, infertility and contraceptive procedures, sex change operations, mental illness and personality disorders, AIDS, drug addiction or alcoholism,

> treatment of injuries arising from direct participation in civil commotion or strikes, and self inflicted injuries.... The significance of this list of exclusions can be appreciated by comparing the list of Medisave exclusions...with the list of National Health Priority Areas (NHPA) in Australia. The NHPA is an initiative of Australia's nine commonwealth, state, and territory governments, and it focuses on "diseases and other conditions that contribute most significantly to Australia's burden of illness and for which there is potential for the burden to be significantly reduced" (Australian Institute of Health and Welfare 1999:93).... The only items on the NHPA list that do not appear on the Medishield list of exclusions are asthma and personal injury (pp. 719–720).

It can be inferred from this passage that by categorically excluding certain procedures, Singapore's health care system affirms a particular concept of basic health care, which Barr's regards as overly narrow. The second of Barr's criticisms can then be summarized as follows:

> Criticism 2: Singapore's Health care system fails to provide all the services that can be categorized as basic health care and to which persons may have a legitimate moral right, but for which resources are not available due to government controls on health care expenditures.

Barr also scrutinizes the family based self-help concept inherent in Singapore's healthcare system. As was noted earlier, funds in one's Medisave account may be used to pay for other family members' medical costs. Barr argues that in the case of persons in the lower class, this tends to have the result of one disadvantaged group subsidizing another disadvantaged group, which Barr takes to be morally problematic (pp. 722–723). Although Barr does not explicitly state it, he apparently holds the view that it is unjust for poor persons to subsidize the health care costs of other poor persons. A basis for this contention would be the view that poor persons should not be forced to pay for the health care costs of their family members because all persons have a moral right to have their basic health care needs met by either the government or those members of society that are not among the least well off. This criticism of Barr's, which may in part be supported by egalitarian commitments, can be summarized as follows:

> Criticism 3: The family based, self-help concept inherent in Singapore's healthcare system as well as the numerous government controls is unjust because it results in members of the least well off class paying for the health care costs of their family members.

4 Analyzing Barr's Criticisms

4.1 Analysis of Criticism 1

> Criticism 1: Singapore's health care system is problematic because of the limits it places on the autonomy of persons in the middle and lower classes.

This criticism presupposes that:

(1) Autonomy is a moral value that should be promoted and respected.
(2) The value of autonomy is not outweighed by other moral values in this context.

While many might regard (1) as being obviously true, it should be noted that there is some disagreement about exactly is meant by autonomy. Autonomy is widely defined in the west as the ability to make rational decisions that are free of excessive, inappropriate influences (Brody, 2002; Savulescu, 1994). Some feminists and persons who ascribe to what might be called an Eastern philosophy define autonomy as the ability to make rational decisions that take into account relations with others that are crucial to one's identity (Mackenzie & Stoljar, 2002; Friedman, 2002; Tao, 2004). There are also many variations of the both the western and eastern conceptions of autonomy. There is also some disagreement about whether autonomy should be regarded as intrinsically valuable or valuable in itself or whether it should be viewed as extrinsically valuable, that is, valuable only insofar as it promotes other values that are intrinsically valuable. Hedonist based utilitarian theories are an example of this latter view; such theories hold that autonomy is valuable only so far as it promotes happiness or pleasure.

Assuming (1) is true, (2) remains a contentious issue in philosophy. Some philosophers have argued that autonomy in most contexts carries considerably more weight than other competing values. Such arguments rely on or presuppose some metric for weighing values that gives autonomy priority over all other values. However, if such a theory holds that *sometimes* another competing value can have more weight in certain instances, then the competing value could provide a compelling reason to pursue that alternative which best promotes that value. For instance, Singapore's health care system could be justified if the value of the long time survival of society in this context carries considerably more weight than the value of autonomy, and Singapore's health care system best promotes survival[2]. Furthermore, there are other theories that rank other values equal to or higher than autonomy. Persons who hold such a theory might argue that Singapore's health care is not morally problematic if (1) it can be shown that such a system best contributes significantly to those values ranked equal to or higher than autonomy and (2) the weight assigned to these outcomes exceeds in this context the weight given to autonomy. Similarly, persons offering theories that hold that autonomy is valuable if it promotes some other some other value, will argue that choosing that alternative which diminishes autonomy is not problematic if that alternative more effectively promotes those outcomes that are intrinsically more valuable. For instance, hedonist utilitarians might hold that Singapore's healthcare system is morally appropriate despite the fact that other systems might better promote the value of autonomy if it can be shown that Singapore's system best promotes happiness.

Before concluding this section, it should be noted that in recent years, certain cultural particularists have given arguments for the view that (Bell, 2000):

(1) Cultural factors can affect how values are ranked.
(2) Cultural factors can affect how moral values are justified.
(3) Cultural factors can provide the moral foundations for distinct political practices and institutions.

The first point is particularly important for this discussion.[3] Many East Asian philosophers have argued that many persons living in countries such as Singapore, which have a Confucian heritage, rank values quite different than many persons living in western countries. Confucianism is a teleological philosophy, which holds that the end of all human action is to bring about the harmony of the universe (Chan, 1963). Furthermore, the harmony of the universe can only be obtained by bringing about the harmony of the society in which one lives, and that this precondition can itself only be realized by making those families who reside there harmonious and this in turn can only occur through personal cultivation. Therefore, the value of societal harmony carries much weight in Confucianism. Many hold that this value continues to influence Asian societies. As Singapore's Lee Kuan Yew states, Singaporeans have "little doubt that a society with communitarian values where the interests of society take precedence over that of the individuals suits them better than the individualism of America" (*International Herald Tribune*, 1991). No doubt, this view is also reflected in the health care system adopted by Singapore.

Therefore, if one wishes to argue that Singapore's health care system is problematic because of the limits it places on the autonomy of persons in the middle and lower classes, one must first defend the value index or basic moral intuitions that support this viewpoint. Moreover, one must show that the weight one gives to these values can be justified by sound rational arguments, which do not rely on culture specific moral intuitions or principles, but rather appeal to basic moral intuitions or principles to which all fully rational persons must agree to.

4.2 Analysis of Criticism 2

> Criticism 2: Singapore's health care system fails to provide all the services that can be categorized as basic health care and to which persons may have a legitimate moral right but for which resources are not available due to government controls on health care expenditures.

This criticism presupposes that:

(1) persons have a legitimate moral right to basic health care against society.
(2) such a right is not trumped by other rights.
(3) some of the services that are not subsidized by Singapore's government would fall under the category of basic health care.

(1) is a positive claim right because the right being asserted has the following form:

> X has a right against Y to provide Z if and only if Y is obligated to provide Z to X (Hohfield, 1919).

There are number of arguments that can be given for (1). This essay, however, will only focus on several of the more substantial and widely cited arguments. One such argument is Norman Daniels' argument from equal opportunity (Daniels, 1982, 1985). Daniels' argument utilizes the principle of fair opportunity given in John Rawls seminal work, *A Theory of Justice*, to argue that all persons have a legitimate right to basic health care. The principle of fair opportunity is one of the three principles of justice that Rawls claims should be used construct and shape the basic structure of society, the "way in which major social institutions fit together into one system, and how they assign fundamental rights and duties and shape the division of advantages that arises through social cooperation" (*Political Liberalism*, 1993, p. 258).

The principle of fair opportunity is roughly the claim that social and economic inequalities are to be arranged so that they are attached to offices and positions open to all under the conditions of fair equality of opportunity. Daniels argues that because a just society is obligated to promote equality of opportunity and because normal human functioning is a necessary condition for enjoying the normal opportunity range in any society, a just society is also obligated to ensure that each of its members is functioning at a normal level. Since disease, disability and other health-related maladies cause humans to function at below a normal level, it, therefore, follows that a just society is obligated to provide enough health care to each of its members to restore basic human functioning.[4]

However, as some philosophers have noted (Wasserman, 1998) a lack of skills and talents also prevents one from enjoying the normal opportunity range. Some have argued that Daniel's argument for why all persons have a right to basic health care also commits him to the claim that society is also obligated to aid those persons whose lack of skills and talents prevent them from them enjoying the normal range. The challenge for proponents of Daniels is to show why society is only obligated to provide some of those goods and services that are necessary to enjoy the normal range and not others.

Liberty or freedom is sometimes also appealed to arguing for why all persons have the right to health care (Green, 1976, 1983). Such arguments tend to have the following structure:

(1) All persons possess civil liberties.
(2) A society should respect civil liberties.
(3) The enjoyment of civil liberties presupposes the possession of a basic set of goods.
(4) Health care is one of those goods that one must possess in order to enjoy civil liberties.
(5) Respect for civil liberties requires society to ensure that all persons have the means necessary to exercise those liberties.
(6) Therefore, a society is obligated to provide health care for all persons.
(7) Therefore, all persons have a right to basic health care against society.

This type of argument is subject to a number of criticisms. First, it presupposes that liberty is a value, which always outranks other values, and this is not a view that is universally shared. As was noted in the case of autonomy, different cultures and moral theories may not regard liberty as always being lexically prior to other values. Second, some might argue that the claim that all persons ought to respect the civil liberties of others does not require society to ensure that all persons have the means necessary to exercise those liberties, but merely that all persons ought to refrain from directly violating persons' liberties.

Another argument, which can be given for why persons have a moral right to basic health care, appeals to the notion of respect for persons. Many philosophers hold the view that we ought to respect persons, those beings who possess certain attributes and are capable of performing certain activities and that one way to respect persons is to ascribe positive claim rights to them (Quinn, 1993). By ascribing positive claim rights to them, we are respecting persons by fostering those conditions that give rise to those activities that are essential for a person. Bearing this in mind, some form of the following value argument might be employed in order to justify the claim that persons have a moral right to basic health care.[5]

(1) Persons are those beings who can perform certain activities and possess certain attributes, which we all regard as intrinsically valuable.
(2) Because we all regard these activities and attributes as intrinsically valuable, we all should respect persons by fostering the conditions that give rise to these activities and attributes.
(3) Normal human functioning is necessary in order to engage in those activities and develop those attributes that we regard as intrinsically valuable.
(4) Therefore, in order to show proper respect for persons, we ought to ensure that all persons have basic health care.
(5) Therefore, all persons have right to basic health care against society.

This value argument as it is presented has undeniably vague premises. Persons giving such an argument must specify the premises and give an argument for which activities and attributes we should regard as intrinsically valuable. However, some might argue that while most individuals may agree that a person can perform certain activities or possess certain attributes that we regard as intrinsically valuable, as was the case in the previous argument, they might define what it means to "respect" persons negatively. That is, there is reason to hold that to respect persons is merely not to interfere with the performance or development of these activities. However, if this is true this argument does not show that a society ought to provide people with basic health care.

In addition to appealing to certain attributes that belong to a person, the claim that persons have certain positive claim rights can also be justified if it can be shown that the general observance of such rights helps to achieve an optimal distribution of interests, and that this overrides other moral considerations (Quinn, 1993).[6] Therefore, according to this argument, if one can argue that ascribing a right to basic health care to all persons helps to achieve an optimal distribution of interests, then one can justify the claim that all persons have such a right. However, such an argument among other things presupposes that there is some optimal distribution of interests that can be obtained and therefore can only succeed if one can show why one should attempt to achieve this particular distribution of interests and not any other distribution of interests. This is a notoriously difficult problem for persons giving consequentialist arguments as there is no shared metric for weighing interests.[7]

Turning now to the second assumption, it should be noted that even if an argument can be made for the claim that all persons have a basic right to health care, many persons subscribe to the notion that many rights can be trumped by other rights (Brody, 2004). That is, when two or more rights conflict with one another,[8] one ought to act in accordance with that right that carries more force in this particular situation. Of course, some rights theorists have also argued that some rights can never trumped. Similarly, many philosophers also hold that certain moral appeals can trump other moral appeals only in a certain context (Brody, 2004); (Nagel, 2002). For instance, depending on the context an appeal to consequences might trump the appeal to rights (Nagel, 2002). It seems then that in order for Barr's criticism to be taken seriously, one must also show that the right to basic health care can (1) never be trumped; (2) that in this context the right to basic health care is not trumped by any other rights; or (3) the right to health care is not trumped by some other moral appeal. Furthermore, as was shown in the previous section, the arguments that one gives for these claims must utilize premises that all rational persons will agree to.

Finally, as was noted in the beginning of this section Barr's argument also presupposes that some of the services that are not subsidized by Singapore's government would fall under the category of basic health care. This presupposition, in turn, presupposes a theory of what constitutes basic health care. One popular theory of what constitutes basic health care ties back to the argument given by Norman Daniels. Basic health care is simply whatever health care is necessary to restore humans to normal human functioning (Daniels, 2000). Unfortunately, there is considerable disagreement about what constitutes normal human functioning.

For instance, Daniels has famously argued that normal human functioning can be determined by examining the design of the organism to determine the "natural functional organization" of its members and by using statistical analysis to determine the statistical average for some realm of human activity. However, as Paul Root Wolpe observes a number of philosophers have argued that it is difficult to determine the "natural functional organization" of humans and that it is, therefore, difficult to identify normal functioning for a number of traits (Wolpe, 2002). Other philosophers have argued that because cultures and ideologies play a strong role in determining which traits are considered typical or normal, it is impossible to "discover" what constitutes normal human functioning (Holstein, 2000; McCrea, 1983; Silvers, 1998).

It is of course possible to advance other explanations for what constitutes basic health care that do not appeal to human functioning. Arguments like the one above assume that we can come to learn what basic health care ought to compass. However, some philosophers who hold argue that this is impossible claim that we should instead appeal to discussion and consent in order to construct a notion of basic health care that takes into account certain values (Engelhardt, 1992). In any event, one can only argue that Singapore's health care system morally fails if it can be shown that Singapore does not subsidize all of the services that fall under a concept of basic health care to which persons have a right.

4.3 Analysis of Criticism 3

> Criticism 3: The family based, self-help concept inherent in Singapore's healthcare system as well as the numerous government controls is unjust because it results in members of the least well off class paying for the health care costs of their family members.

This criticism presupposes that:

> Those that the least well off have a moral right to have their basic health care needs met by either the government or those members of society that are not among the least well off.

The arguments that can be used to justify the claim that all persons have a right to basic health care against society can also be used to justify this presupposition. In addition, it can also be argued that the difference principle, one of the other principles of justice given in Rawls's theory of justice, supports this claim. The difference principle states that social and economic inequalities in a society are to be to the greatest benefit of the least advantaged members of society (*Theory of Justice*, 1971, p. 302). This is roughly the claim that if it is possible to raise the absolute position of the least advantaged further by having some inequalities of income and wealth, then we ought to promote inequality until the absolute position of the least advantaged can no longer be raised.

Using this claim as a foundation, one could argue that because social and economic inequalities in a society are to be to the greatest benefit of the least well off, this entails that society is obligated to provide the poor with free basic health care in most instances.[9] Further argumentation is, of course, necessary to show how free basic health care is to the greatest benefit of the least well off. One must also define what one means by "benefit." One must also justify a particular ranking of values in order to show that free basic health care produces the desired effect of being to the greatest benefit of the least well off.

One can only secure this argument if one accepts the difference principle. However, many philosophers argue that the difference principle is irreparably problematic and should be abandoned. Consequentialists argue that acting in accordance with the difference principle may not always yield the best state of affairs.[10] Others argue that the difference principle ignores principles of desert. Such persons adhere to one or more of the following principles:

(a) People should be rewarded for their work activity based on what they contribute to the social product (Miller, 1976; Miller, 1989; Riley, 1989).

(b) People should be rewarded based on the effort they expend while working (Lamont, 1995).

(c) People should be rewarded based on the costs they incurred while working (Sadurski, 1985; Lamont, 1997).

Such persons argue that the difference principle ignores claims that argue that (1) because of their hard work and contributions some persons deserve a higher level of material goods even if this does not improve the absolute position of the least well off and (2) the Difference Principle does not take into account how persons end up among the least well off. A person who adheres to the difference principle must address these objections.

Libertarians on the other hand argue that the difference principle may involve the immoral takings of just holdings. Libertarians hold that a distribution of resources is just if everyone is entitled to whatever they possess irrespective of their needs (Nozick, 1974). A person is justly entitled to *whatever* she acquires so long as she acts in accordance with the principle of just acquisition or the principle of just transfer. Ownership is not reducible to fairness making conditions. It is important to understand that many libertarians regard property as an extension of persons so that (1) persons have a right to freely distribute their goods as they please and (2) goods can only be transferred from one party to another if both the parties agree to this exchange. Consequently, libertarians regard market rationing as justified and hold that taxation may be unjustified if it is used to pay for services for which one has not consented to pay for. According to the difference principle, however, persons *only* have a right to a greater level of material goods than others if the possession of that right improves the position of the least well off. This suggests that persons may be required to relinquish some of their holdings to raise the absolute position of the least well off even if they acted in accordance with the principle of just acquisition or the principle of just transfer when acquiring their holdings.

It is interesting to note that Singapore's government does recognize property rights as central to a person's identity. For instance, persons are allowed to purchase whatever healthcare they please, which is not the case in countries with an egalitarian health care system such as the one found in Canada. Singapore's government however, should not be regarded as being perfectly congruent with a libertarian account. Libertarians hold that persons are allowed to do as they please so long as they do not infringe upon other's rights. However, in Singapore, certain civil liberties are restricted and persons through taxation are forced to pay for services to which they have not agreed. Finally, libertarians regard the state as an institution whose soul duty is to protect the life and property rights of its citizens; Singapore, which claims a much broader compass of authorities, treats the state as though it were a community.

One last objection that should be considered and that has attracted some attention in recent years is the communitarian argument that standards of justice vary depending on context and must be found in the in the traditions and forms of life of particular societies (Mackie, 1978; Benhabib, 1992; Macintyre, 1978; Sandel, 1998; Taylor, 1985, 1999; Walzer, 1983). In contrast, the Difference Principle and the other principles of justice given by Rawls are principles that are regarded by many as universally true. However, communitarians argue that moral judgments will depend on the particular interpretive framework and language of reasons within which agents view their world (Benhabib, 1992; Macintyre, 1978; Sandel, 1998; Taylor, 1985, 1999). Further, Michael Walzer argues that even if universal moral principles can be derived by abstracting away beliefs, practices ,and institutions that influence our perspective of the world, "any set [of universal principles] would have to be considered in terms so abstract that they would be of little use in thinking about particular distributions" (Walzer, 1983, p. 8).

Adherence to communitarianism might lead us to embrace societal specific standards of justice. As was noted, some scholars have argued that Singapore has been heavily influenced by a Confucian ethos. According to Confucianism, a just society is a harmonious society and a harmonious society is one inhabited by *ren* persons. To be a *ren* person is to be a moral individual who has fully cultivated all of the separate virtues to the highest degree (Schwartz; Waley; Van Norden) and who expresses the type of affection that is appropriate given one's role in a particular relationship. It is also commonly though that a harmonious society is one where people learn the virtue of *ren* by taking care of each other:

> In the field of a district, those who belong to the same nine squares render all friendly offices to one another in their going out and coming in, aid one another in keeping watch and ward, and sustain one another in sickness. Thus, the people are brought together to live in affection and harmony (Mencius, 3A:3:18).

In this passage, the local community and not the government is claimed to bear primary responsibility for providing healthcare to persons.

According to such an ethos, the family based self-help concept inherent in Singapore's healthcare system as well as the numerous government controls are not seen as unjust to members of the least well off class. Rather, the whole system is seen as just. By encouraging families to provide for their members health care needs, persons are able to express the type of affection that is appropriate given their role in a particular relationship, and which is necessary to be a *ren* person. Further, such actions promote the harmony of the family, which in turn contributes to the harmony of the state.

There is, of course, some debate about how ingrained Confucian values are in Singapore's culture. However, if this is indeed the case and communitarianism is a defensible view, then it can be argued that to claim that such a system is unjust is simply false.

5 Conclusion

This essay considered three moral criticisms that were raised against Singapore's health care system by Michael T. Barr. There is a sense in which the considerations raised by Barr against Singapore's health care system are not unique to Singapore. Other health care systems are often criticized for placing unacceptable limits on persons' autonomy, for failing to provide the appropriate scope of free basic care to all persons and for being unjust to those among the least well off. As should be apparent from this essay, all of the arguments given by Barr rely on presuppositions, which (1) may not be intuitively obvious to many persons and (2) may not be universally agreed upon.

If one is to argue that Singapore's health care system places unacceptable limits on autonomy, after defining autonomy, one must show that no competing moral values outrank the value of autonomy. This is no easy task, as one must also show that one's ranking of values is not merely a product of one's culture, but is justifiable using some universally shared reasons. This challenge bears against all of Barr's criticisms of Singapore. Persons wishing to endorse all of Barr's criticisms have the burden of giving additional arguments in support of the assumptions that underlie his criticisms, and these arguments in turn must not utilize premises that rely on culture-specific intuitions.

In addition, if one is to argue that Singapore's health care system fails to provide all of the services that can be categorized as basic health care and to which persons may have a legitimate moral right, one must first show that some argument can be given for why persons have such right. However, as was noted in this essay, many of the arguments that have often been given in support of such claims face a number of difficult criticisms. One must show why the right to health care is not trumped by other rights, moral appeals, or values. In particular, one must respond to the consequentialist claim that Singapore's system best promotes the long term well being of a society as a whole. One must also show that the services not provided by Singapore's health care system fall under a concept of basic health care that we have reason to accept.

Finally, if one claims that Singapore's health care system is unjust because the family based self- help concept inherent in Singapore's healthcare system leads poor persons to pay for the health care costs of their family members, one must also show why persons among the least well off have a right to basic health care. In doing so, one must address the objections of certain consequentialists, persons who adhere to certain desert based principles, as well as libertarians, all of whom argue that none are only some of those persons from among the least well off are entitled to free basic health care.

This is not to say that arguments like Barr's carry no force at all, or should be dismissed. It is important to reiterate that the intent of this essay was not to defend Singapore's health care system against Barr's criticisms, but merely to analyze these criticisms from a philosophical perspective. The above analysis, however, shows that until strong philosophical arguments can be given in support Barr's criticisms, there always will be some degree of doubt about whether we are justified in making such moral judgments.

6 Appendix

Table 1 Chart A: Percentage of GDP spent on health care

Country	1998	1999	2000	2001	2002
United States	13.0	13.0	13.1	13.9	14.6
Canada	9.2	9.0	8.9	9.4	9.6
United Kingdom	6.9	7.2	7.3	7.5	7.7
China	4.8	5.1	5.6	5.7	5.8
Hong Kong	4.8	5.6	5.5	5.5	5.7
Singapore	4.2	4.1	3.6	3.9	4.3

Source: World Health Organization (2005); Hong Kong Department of Health (2003/2004)

Table 2 Chart B: Government expenditure on health as % of total expenditure of health

Country	1998	1999	2000	2001	2002
United Kingdom	80.4	80.6	80.9	83.0	83.4
Canada	70.6	70.3	70.4	70.1	69.9
United States	44.5	44.3	44.4	44.9	44.9
China	39.0	38.0	34.6	35.5	33.7
Hong Kong	51.0	55.0	56.0	56.0	57.0
Singapore	41.6	38.3	35.2	33.5	30.9

Source: World Health Organization (2005); Hong Kong Department of Health (2003/2004)

Table 3 Chart C: Private expenditure on health as % of total expenditure of health

Country	1998	1999	2000	2001	2002
United States	55.5	55.7	55.6	55.1	55.1
Canada	29.4	29.7	29.6	29.9	30.1
United Kingdom	19.6	19.4	19.1	17.0	16.6
China	61.0	62.0	65.4	64.5	66.3
Hong Kong	49.0	45.0	44.0	44.0	43.0
Singapore	58.4	61.7	64.8	66.5	69.1

Source: World Health Organization (2005); Hong Kong Department of Health (2003/2004)

Table 4 Chart D: Out of pocket expenditure as % of private expenditure on health

Country	1998	1999	2000	2001	2002
United States	28.0	27.6	27.1	26.2	25.4
Canada	55.2	55.1	53.7	51	50.3
United Kingdom	55.7	55.2	54.7	58.1	55.9
China	94	94.9	95.6	95.7	96.3
Hong Kong	35	31	33	31	30
Singapore	97.3	97.4	97.2	97	97.3

Source: World Health Organization (2005); Hong Kong Department of Health (2003/2004)

Acknowledgments I would like to thank H. Tristram Engelhardt, Jr. and Chris Ralston for all their helpful comments.

Notes

1 The CPF contribution rates are revisable according to the economy, age group and whether one is in the public or private sector. At one time when the economy was doing very well, the contribution rate for both employee and employer was as high as 20%. For a more detailed breakdown of CPF contribution rates, see Central Provident Fund website at http://www.cpf.gov.sg/cpf_info/Online/contrira.asp

[2] In his speech, "Can Good Healthcare be cheap or even free?", Wan, Khaw Boon (2006), Singapore's Minister for health, argued that Singapore's health care system has to ration and implement the controls that it does if it wishes to publicly finance health care and be financially sustainable in the long.

[3] For a more in depth discussion of Communitarianism, see David Bell's "Communitarianism" (1997), in *The Blackwell Encyclopedic Dictionary of Business Ethics*, Prentice Hall, and *Communitarianism and Its Critics* (1993).

[4] This is the view held most notably by Norman Daniels (1985).

[5] Gutman gives a version of this argument in her essay "For and Against Equal Access Health Care" (1981).

[6] This is the view commonly attributed to consequentialists. J.S. Mill (1998) describes this view in his seminal work *Utilitarianism*.

[7] See *Utilitarianism and Its Critics,* (1990) for more in-depth criticisms against consequentialism.

[8] Sinnott-Armstrong (1996) gives an excellent account of how rights may conflict in "Moral Dilemmas and Rights".

[9] Alastair Campbell and others (1997) have noted that the Difference principle must only require that an economically challenged country may only have to provide very limited health care if any further attempt to raise the level of free health care would hamper economic development and make the worse off even more worse off.

[10] For a more in depth discussion and analysis of how consequentialists think goods should be distributed, see Nicholas Rescher's *Distributive Justice: A Constructive Critique of the Utilitarian Theory of Distribution* (1966).

References

Barr, M. (2001). Medical savings accounts in Singapore: A critical inquiry. *Journal of Health Politics, Policy and Law, 26*(4), 709–726.

Bell, D. (1993). *Communitarianism and its critics*. Oxford: Clarendon Press

Bell, D. (1997). Communitarianism. In P. H. Werhane and R. E. Freeman (Eds.), *The Blackwell encyclopedic dictionary of business ethics*. Prentice Hall Malden: Blackwell.

Bell, D. (2000). *East meets west: Human rights and democracy in East Asia*. Princeton: Princeton University Press

Benhabib, S. (1992). *Situating the self: Gender, community and postmodernism in contemporary ethics*. Cambridge: Polity Press.

Brody, B. (2002). Making informed consent meaningful. *IRB: Ethics and Human Research, 23*(5), 1–5.

Brody, B. (2004). *Taking issue: Pluralism and casuistry in bioethics*. Washington DC: Georgetown University Press.

Campbell, A., Gillett, G., & Jones, G. (1997). *Medical ethics* (2nd ed.). Auckland: Oxford University Press.

Chan, W. (1963). *A source book in Chinese philosophy*. Princeton: Princeton University Press.

Daniels, N. (1982). Equality of access to healthcare. *MMFQ, 60*(1), Milbank Memorial Fund.

Daniels, N. (1985). *Just health care*. Cambridge: Cambridge University Press.

Daniels, N. (2000). Normal human functioning and the treatment enhancement distinction. *Cambridge Quarterly, 9*(3), 309–322.

Engelhardt, H. T., Jr. (1992). Why a two-tier system of health care delivery is morally unavoidable. In A. Strosberg, J. Wiener, R. Baker, & I. Fein (Eds.), *Rationing America's medical care: The Oregon plan and beyond*. Washington, DC: Brookings Institute.

Friedman, M. (2002). Autonomy, social disruption, and women. In C. MacKenzie & N. Stoljar (Eds.), *Relational autonomy: Feminist perspectives on autonomy, agency and the social self.* Oxford: Oxford University Press.

Glover, J. (Ed.). (1990). *Utilitarianism and its critics*. New York: Macmillan Publishing Company.

Green, R. (1976). Health care and justice in contract theory perspective. In R. Veatch & R. Branson (Eds.), *Ethics and health policy*. Cambridge: Ballinger.
Green, R. (1983). The priority of health care. *Journal of Medicine and Philosophy, 8*, 373–80.
Gutman, A. (1981). For and against equal access health care, *MMFQ, 59*(4), Milbank Memorial Fund.
Hohfield, W. (1919). *Fundamental legal conceptions*. In W. Cook (Ed.). New Haven: Yale University Press.
Holstein, M. (2000). Aging, culture, and the framing of Alzheimer disease. In P. Whitehouse, K. Maurer, & J. Ballenger (Eds.), *Concepts of Alzheimer disease: Biological, clinical and cultural perspectives*. Baltimore: John Hopkins University Press.
Hong Kong Department of Health Annual Report. (2003/2004). [Online]. Available: http://www.info.gov.hk/dh/publicat/ar0304/start.swf. Accessed July 22, 2005
Lamont, J. (1997). Incentive income, deserved income, and economic rents. *Journal of Political Philosophy, 5*, 26–46
Lamont, J. (1995). Problems for effort-based distribution principles. *Journal of Applied Philosophy, 12*, 215–229
Low, L. (1998). Health care in the context of social security in Singapore. *SOJOURN: Journal of Social Issues in Southeast Asia, 13*, 139–165.
MacIntyre, A. (1978). *Against the self-images of the age*. Notre Dame: University of Notre Dame Press
MacKenzie, C., & Stoljar, N. (Eds.). (2002). *Autonomy refigured, relational autonomy: Feminist perspectives on autonomy, agency, and the social self* (pp. 3–31). Oxford: Oxford University Press.
Mackie, J. L. (1978). *Ethics: Inventing right and wrong*. London: Penguin Books.
Massaro, T., & Wong, Y. (1995). Positive experience with medical savings accounts in Singapore. *Health Affairs, 14*, 267–269.
McCrea, F. (1983). The politics of menopause: The 'discovery' of a deficiency disease. *Social Problems, 31*(1), 111–123.
Mencius (2003). *Mencius*. D.C. Lau (trans.). Hong Kong: The Chinese University Press.
Mill, J.S. (1998). *Utilitarianism*. Edited with an introduction by Roger Crisp. New York: Oxford University Press. Originally published in 1861.
Miller, D. (1976). *Social justice*. Oxford: Clarendon Press.
Miller, D. (1989). *Market, state, and community*. Oxford: Clarendon Press.
Ministry of Health. (1999). *Report of the cost review committee-response of the Ministry of Health*. [On-line]. Available: http://gov.sg/moh/mohiss/review.html.
Nagel, T. (2002). *Concealment and exposure*. Oxford: Oxford University Press.
Nozick, R. (1974). *Anarchy, state and Utopia*. New York: Basic Books.
Ramsay, C. (2001). Beyond the public-private debate: An examination of quality, access and cost in the health care systems of eight countries, prepared by Western Sky Communication [Vancouver] for Marigold Foundation. Calgary: Canada.
Rawls, J. (1971). *A theory of justice*. Harvard, MA: Harvard University Press.
Rawls, J. (1993). *Political liberalism*. New York: Columbia University Press.
Rescher, N. (1966). *Distributive justice: A constructive critique of the utilitarian theory of distribution*. Indianapolis: Bobbs-Merrill Co.
Riley, J. (1989). Justice under capitalism. In J. W. Chapman (Ed.), *Markets and justice* (pp. 122–162). New York: New York University Press.
Sadurski, W. (1985). *Giving desert its due*. Dordrecht, Holland: D. Reidel.
Sinnott-Armstrong, W. (1996). Moral dilemmas and rights. In H. E. Mason (Ed.), *Moral dilemmas and moral theory* (pp. 48–65). New York: Oxford University Press.
Silvers, A. (1998). A Fatal attraction to normalizing, treating disabilities as deviations from species typical human functioning. In E. Parens (Ed.), *Enhancing human traits* (pp 95–123). Washington, DC: Georgetown University Press.
Sandel, M. (1998). *Liberalism and the limits of justice* (2nd ed.). Cambridge: Cambridge University Press.

Savulescu, J. (1994). Rational desires and the limitation of life sustaining treatment. *Bioethics, 8*(3), 191–122.
Tan, M & Chew, B. (1997). *Affordable health care: Issues and prospects.* Singapore: Prentice Hall.
Taylor, C. (1985). *Philosophy and the human sciences: philosophical papers 2.* Cambridge: Cambridge University Press.
Taylor, C. (1999). Conditions of an unforced consensus on human rights. In J. R. Bauer & D. Bell (Eds.), *The East Asian challenge for human rights.* New York: Cambridge University Press.
Tao, J. (2004). Confucian and western notion of human need and agency: Health care and biomedical ethics in the twenty-first century. In R. Qui (Ed.), *Asian bioethics.* Dordrecht: Kluwer Academic Publishers.
Tucci, J. (2004, October). The Singapore health system – achieving positive health outcomes with low expenditure. *Health Market Review.* [On-line]. Available: watsonwyatt.com/europe/pubs/healthcare/render2.asp?ID=13850
Quinn, W. (1993). *Morality and action.* Cambridge: Cambridge University Press.
Van Norden, B. (2002). Introduction. In B. Van Norden (Ed.), *Confucius and the Analects.* New York: Oxford University Press.
Waley, A. (1989). *The Analects of Confucius.* New York: First Vintage Books.
Walzer, M. (1983). *Spheres of justice.* Oxford: Blackwell.
Wan, K. B. (2006). *Can good healthcare be cheap or even free? Ministry of Health.* [On-line]. Available: http://www.moh.gov.sg/corp/about/newsroom/speeches/details.do?id=36470793. Accessed June 29, 2006.
Wasserman, D. (1998). Distributive justice. In A. Wasserman, D. Mahowald, M. B. Becker, L. C. Silvers (Eds.), *Disability, difference, discrimination: Perspectives on justice in Bioethics and public policy (Point/Counterpoint).* New York: Roman Littlefield.
Wolpe, P. (2002). Treatment, enhancement and the ethics of neurotherapeutics. *Brain and Cognition, 50*, 387–95.
World Bank. (2003). *Is Singapore a model for health financing?* [On-line]. Available: http://rru.worldbank.org/Discussions/Discussion.aspx?id=23. Accessed April 25, 2006.
World Health Organization. (2005). *World health report* 2005. [Online]. Available: http://www.who.int/hrh/about_whr05/en/. Accessed July 19, 2005.
Yew, L. K. (1991, 9–10 November). Quoted in the *International Herald Tribune.*

Index